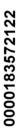

IT HAPPENED TO ME

Series Editor: Arlene Hirschfelder

Books in the It Happened to Me series are designed for inquisitive teens digging for answers about certain illnesses, social issues, or lifestyle interests. Whether you are deep into your teen years or just entering them, these books are gold mines of up-to-date information, riveting teen views, and great visuals to help you figure out stuff. Besides special boxes highlighting singular facts, each book is enhanced with the latest reading lists, websites, and an index. Perfect for browsing, there are loads of expert information by acclaimed writers to help parents, guardians, and librarians understand teen illness, tough situations, and lifestyle choices.

1. *Epilepsy: The Ultimate Teen Guide,* by Kathlyn Gay and Sean McGarrahan, 2002.
2. *Stress Relief: The Ultimate Teen Guide,* by Mark Powell, 2002.
3. *Learning Disabilities: The Ultimate Teen Guide,* by Penny Hutchins Paquette and Cheryl Gerson Tuttle, 2003.
4. *Making Sexual Decisions: The Ultimate Teen Guide,* by L. Kris Gowen, 2003.
5. *Asthma: The Ultimate Teen Guide,* by Penny Hutchins Paquette, 2003.
6. *Cultural Diversity—Conflicts and Challenges: The Ultimate Teen Guide,* by Kathlyn Gay, 2003.
7. *Diabetes: The Ultimate Teen Guide,* by Katherine J. Moran, 2004.
8. *When Will I Stop Hurting? Teens, Loss, and Grief: The Ultimate Teen Guide to Dealing with Grief,* by Ed Myers, 2004.
9. *Volunteering: The Ultimate Teen Guide,* by Kathlyn Gay, 2004.
10. *Organ Transplants—A Survival Guide for the Entire Family: The Ultimate Teen Guide,* by Tina P. Schwartz, 2005.
11. *Medications: The Ultimate Teen Guide,* by Cheryl Gerson Tuttle, 2005.
12. *Image and Identity—Becoming the Person You Are: The Ultimate Teen Guide,* by L. Kris Gowen and Molly C. McKenna, 2005.
13. *Apprenticeship: The Ultimate Teen Guide,* by Penny Hutchins Paquette, 2005.
14. *Cystic Fibrosis: The Ultimate Teen Guide,* by Melanie Ann Apel, 2006.
15. *Religion and Spirituality in America: The Ultimate Teen Guide,* by Kathlyn Gay, 2006.
16. *Gender Identity: The Ultimate Teen Guide,* by Cynthia L. Winfield, 2007.

17. *Physical Disabilities: The Ultimate Teen Guide,* by Denise Thornton, 2007.
18. *Money—Getting It, Using It, and Avoiding the Traps: The Ultimate Teen Guide,* by Robin F. Brancato, 2007.
19. *Self-Advocacy: The Ultimate Teen Guide,* by Cheryl Gerson Tuttle and JoAnn Augeri Silva, 2007.
20. *Adopted: The Ultimate Teen Guide,* by Suzanne Buckingham Slade, 2007.
21. *The Military and Teens: The Ultimate Teen Guide,* by Kathlyn Gay, 2008.
22. *Animals and Teens: The Ultimate Teen Guide,* by Gail Green, 2009.
23. *Reaching Your Goals: The Ultimate Teen Guide,* by Anne Courtright, 2009.
24. *Juvenile Arthritis: The Ultimate Teen Guide,* by Kelly Rouba, 2009.
25. *Obsessive-Compulsive Disorder: The Ultimate Teen Guide,* by Natalie Rompella, 2009.
26. *Body Image and Appearance: The Ultimate Teen Guide,* by Kathlyn Gay, 2009.
27. *Writing and Publishing: The Ultimate Teen Guide,* by Tina P. Schwartz, 2010.
28. *Food Choices: The Ultimate Teen Guide,* by Robin F. Brancato, 2010.
29. *Immigration: The Ultimate Teen Guide,* by Tatyana Kleyn, 2011.
30. *Living with Cancer: The Ultimate Teen Guide,* by Denise Thornton, 2011.
31. *Living Green: The Ultimate Teen Guide,* by Kathlyn Gay, 2012.
32. *Social Networking: The Ultimate Teen Guide,* by Jenna Obee, 2012.
33. *Sports: The Ultimate Teen Guide,* by Gail Fay, 2013.
34. *Adopted: The Ultimate Teen Guide, Revised Edition,* by Suzanne Buckingham Slade, 2013.
35. *Bigotry and Intolerance: The Ultimate Teen Guide,* by Kathlyn Gay, 2013.
36. *Substance Abuse: The Ultimate Teen Guide,* by Sheri Bestor, 2013.
37. *LGBTQ Families: The Ultimate Teen Guide,* by Eva Apelqvist, 2013.
38. *Bullying: The Ultimate Teen Guide,* by Mathangi Subramanian, 2014.
39. *Eating Disorders: The Ultimate Teen Guide,* by Jessica R. Greene, 2014.
40. *Speech and Language Challenges: The Ultimate Teen Guide,* by Marlene Targ Brill, 2014.
41. *Divorce: The Ultimate Teen Guide,* by Kathlyn Gay, 2014.
42. *Depression: The Ultimate Teen Guide,* by Tina P. Schwartz, 2014.
43. *Creativity: The Ultimate Teen Guide,* by Aryna Ryan, 2015.
44. *Shyness: The Ultimate Teen Guide,* by Bernardo J. Carducci, Ph.D, and Lisa Kaiser, 2015.
45. *Food Allergies: The Ultimate Teen Guide,* by Jessica Reino, 2015.

FOOD ALLERGIES

THE ULTIMATE TEEN GUIDE

JESSICA REINO

IT HAPPENED TO ME, NO. 45

ROWMAN & LITTLEFIELD
Lanham • Boulder • New York • London

Published by Rowman & Littlefield
A wholly owned subsidiary of The Rowman & Littlefield Publishing Group, Inc.
4501 Forbes Boulevard, Suite 200, Lanham, Maryland 20706
www.rowman.com

Unit A, Whitacre Mews, 26-34 Stannary Street, London SE11 4AB

British Library Cataloguing in Publication Information Available

Library of Congress Cataloging-in-Publication Data

Reino, Jessica, 1982–
    Food allergies : the ultimate teen guide / Jessica Reino.
        pages cm. — (It happened to me ; no. 45)
    Includes bibliographical references.
    ISBN 978-1-4422-3573-1 (hardback : alk. paper) — ISBN 978-1-4422-3574-8 (ebook)
    1. Food allergy—Juvenile literature. 2. Teenagers—Health and hygiene—Juvenile literature.
    I. Title.
    RC596.R44 2015
    616.9700835—dc23

                                                                              2014049727

♾™ The paper used in this publication meets the minimum requirements of American National Standard for Information Sciences—Permanence of Paper for Printed Library Materials, ANSI/NISO Z39.48-1992.

Printed in the United States of America

To my family,
especially my husband, Kevin, and my children, Richard and Nicholas.
They inspire me every day, and it is because of them that
I am able to live a fulfilling life with food allergies.

Also to all those suffering from food allergies.
I hope that they, too, will not let their food allergies stop them from
being their best selves and living life to the fullest.

Contents

Acknowledgments   ix

Introduction   xi

1   What Are Food Allergies and Why Should You Care
    about Them?   1

2   The Art of Calm-municating: Becoming a Self-Advocate   15

3   Family: From Harshest Critics to Biggest Cheerleaders   29

4   Friend or Frenemy?   41

5   Parties and Athletics   51

6   Creating Your Crew   63

7   Love in the Time of Food Allergies   83

8   Dining In or Out?   93

9   Your Home Away from Home   101

10 The Importance of Reading Labels   119

11 Top Chef: Cooking Well and Living Well with
    Dietary Restrictions   127

Glossary   147

Notes   149

Food Allergy Resources for Teens   157

Index   163

About The Author   167

Acknowledgments

I am so fortunate that I was given the opportunity to write this book and I could not have done so without the assistance and support of many people. I first would like to thank my family. To my husband, Kevin, thank you for supporting me through my journey with food allergies and everything else that comes our way. To my parents, sister, and brother, I would not be where I am today without you. Thank you for everything. To my mother-in-law, father-in-law, and sister-in-law, thank you for all of your support. To my friends, thank you for always being there for me, especially being in my corner when it comes to advocating for me and raising food allergy awareness.

To Dr. David Stukus, Sloane Miller, and Kristin Beltaos, a special thank you for allowing me to interview you for this book and for sharing your knowledge with others in the food allergy community on a daily basis. Your work is greatly appreciated!

Thank you to all of those at Food Allergy Research & Education, the Food Allergy & Anaphylaxis Connection Team, and the Asthma and Allergy Foundation of America New England Chapter for speaking to me about this project and for all the education, awareness, and support you provide for the food allergy community.

A big thank you to all of those teenagers and their families I interviewed for this book. I truly appreciate you taking the time to share your personal stories, and I hope you find this book informative and helpful.

To my editor, Arlene Hirschfelder, thank you for all of your suggestions, advice, and constant encouragement. You have taught me so much about publishing that I will be forever grateful for. Last, but by no means least, a huge thank you to my wonderful agent, Jodell Sadler. Thank you for believing in me and connecting with my writing from the very start. This project never would have happened without you, and I look forward to many more projects in the future!

Introduction

Food is an important aspect to life. Without food, the body would not be able to sustain itself. Food is also an important part of world culture. It brings family and friends together, and business meetings are conducted over lunch and dinner. Colors of caramel and yellow have become synonymous with certain foods—caramel highlights, lemon-yellow shoes, and so on. There is an entire network dedicated to food, and primetime television has also jumped on the bandwagon with such shows as *Top Chef* and *Hell's Kitchen*. Dieting and fads have become part of a billion-dollar industry, but although these diets are trying to get people to eat healthier and lose weight, they are still geared around the food itself. Preparing and eating food is simply part of being human. However, for fifteen million Americans suffering from food allergies, food can be both a great comfort and a catalyst for fear and anxiety.

Life can get hectic for all of us no matter who we are, where we live, or what we do. If you are someone suffering from food allergies, more often than not, life can become a perpetual state of dealing with difficulty after difficulty that can turn into chaos. For a teenager, this can be even more complicated. As a teenager, you are trying to establish yourself as an individual. As a teenager who also happens to have food allergies, you may be receiving more pushback in trying to attain your individuality because of your food allergies. Maybe you have

Food Allergy Statistics

- About three million people in the United States have a peanut and tree nut allergy.
- Two teens in every classroom will have some type of food allergy.
- U.S. Centers for Disease Control reported that allergic reactions account for more than three hundred thousand ambulatory visits for children eighteen and under in the United States.
- Every three minutes, someone is taken to the emergency room as a result of an allergic reaction.
- Epinephrine is the only treatment for someone during an allergic reaction.[a]

> ## Discovery of Epinephrine
>
> In 1897, John Jacob Abel isolated a new compound that was secreted from adrenal glands and gave it the name *epinephrine*, but it was a chemist named Jockichi Takamine who, in 1901, isolated the pure form of the chemical to be used as treatment in an allergic/asthmatic reaction.[b]

been dealing with food allergies all of your life, but never really gave it a thought because your parents or guardians have always been your advocates or provided safe foods. Maybe you are someone who just got diagnosed and feels overwhelmed with the idea that you will need to change your lifestyle, or maybe you are just learning that those foods that didn't agree with you growing up and caused an in-

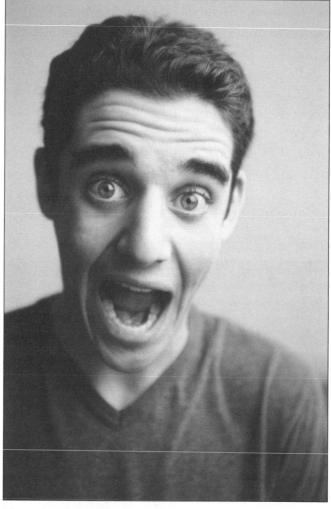

Managing food allergies on your own can be scary, but don't worry—you can do it!

Check This Out: Documentary on Food Allergies

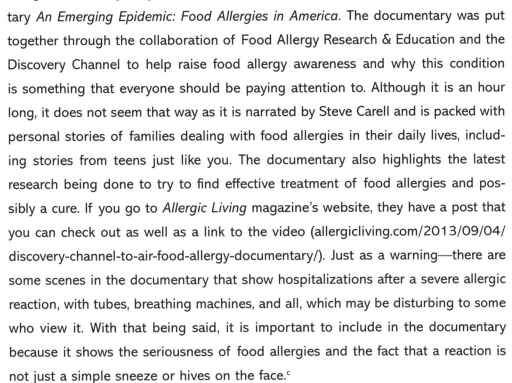

To get an interesting and great overview of living with food allergies and everything it entails, check out the documentary *An Emerging Epidemic: Food Allergies in America*. The documentary was put together through the collaboration of Food Allergy Research & Education and the Discovery Channel to help raise food allergy awareness and why this condition is something that everyone should be paying attention to. Although it is an hour long, it does not seem that way as it is narrated by Steve Carell and is packed with personal stories of families dealing with food allergies in their daily lives, including stories from teens just like you. The documentary also highlights the latest research being done to try to find effective treatment of food allergies and possibly a cure. If you go to *Allergic Living* magazine's website, they have a post that you can check out as well as a link to the video (allergicliving.com/2013/09/04/ discovery-channel-to-air-food-allergy-documentary/). Just as a warning—there are some scenes in the documentary that show hospitalizations after a severe allergic reaction, with tubes, breathing machines, and all, which may be disturbing to some who view it. With that being said, it is important to include in the documentary because it shows the seriousness of food allergies and the fact that a reaction is not just a simple sneeze or hives on the face.[c]

convenient itching sensation are now causing more severe reactions, necessitating you to carry around epinephrine at all times.

How will you manage it on your own? I wish I could tell you that I have it all figured out. I wish I could say that there is some pill you can pop or some magical tonic that you can drink to make it go away at least for a little while. The truth is, I can't. What I can tell you is how I have learned (and continue to learn each day) how to deal with multiple food allergies and to lead a fulfilling life. Other teenagers just like you will offer their tips and advice on what works for them in managing their food allergies. Just like an allergic reaction in which each person's threshold for eating food poses different allergic responses, everyone deals with his or her allergies differently. However, we can all learn from each other and continue to support one another. We can raise awareness, and educate those who are not familiar with this condition because unfortunately, all allergies are on the rise, including food, environmental, and seasonal. The Asthma and Allergy Foundation of America also points out that allergies are a common, yet often overlooked, disease. With allergies being the most frequently reported chronic condition among American children, it's time to pay attention.

WHAT ARE FOOD ALLERGIES AND WHY SHOULD YOU CARE ABOUT THEM?

Now that I have caught your attention regarding the issue of food allergies, are you curious to find out more about them? If not, then you should be. Obviously, if you are suffering from food allergies yourself or if you have a loved one suffering from them, you will be interested in reading more. However, even if you are not familiar with this issue yourself or if you have never experienced food allergies within your own family, there is no denying that they are on the rise. What this means for you is that people with food allergies walk among you on a daily basis. They could be your neighbors, your classmates, your teammates, your coworkers, or even your friends or a romantic partner you have not met yet. Additionally, as you grow older and start your own family, food allergies should be something that you are aware of as they do indeed affect so many children. Many schools are now nut free and have allergy protocols in place, and if you are around these children, you need to be aware of the issue of food allergies.

Food Allergies in History

Although food allergies seem to be a new trend, they have been around for quite some time. In an account from Sir Thomas More, in the late 1400s, when King Henry III broke out into hives after eating strawberries brought to him by Sir William Hastings, the king ordered Hastings beheaded, claiming it was a curse.[a]

First Written Documentation of Food Allergies

In 50 BC, the Roman philosopher Lucretius noted that "what is food for some may be fierce poison for others."[b]

Allergies and Allergic Reactions

So what exactly are food allergies? The National Institute of Allergy and Infectious Diseases defines them as an "abnormal response to food, triggered by the body's immune system."[1] In most cases involving an allergic reaction, the body sees the food as a threat and produces an antibody called immunoglobulin E (IgE), that attaches to certain particles in the food protein and triggers an immune response. While many allergic reactions are IgE mediated, food allergic reactions can also be non-IgE mediated, which means that the reaction occurs

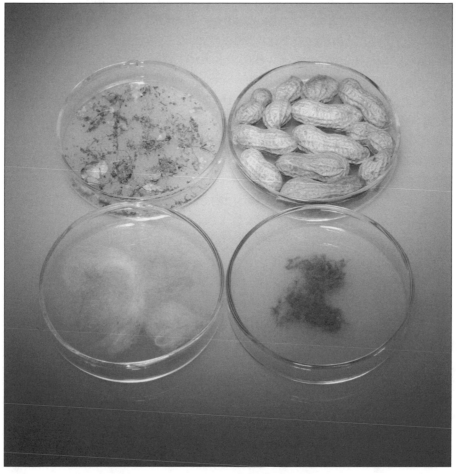

Some examples of foods that can cause an allergic reaction.

The Top Eight

Although any food can be a culprit for a food allergic reaction, the eight major food allergens that are recognized in the United States are peanut, tree nut, soy, wheat, fish, shellfish, milk, and egg. These foods account for 90 percent of food allergic reactions in the United States.[c]

because the food is still seen as a threat by the immune system, but it is not caused by a reaction to the IgE antibody. Really what it boils down to is that a food allergy is an allergic reaction involving the immune system in which the symptoms of a food allergic reaction are reproducible with each and every exposure to that particular food.[2]

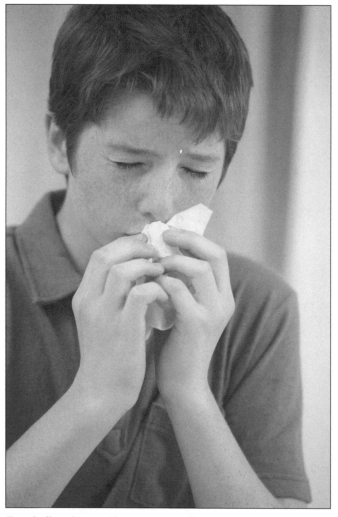

Food allergic reactions cause more than just a sneeze.

It is important to recognize the signs and symptoms of a food allergic reaction. It is far more than a sneeze. The symptoms of a true food allergy can range from mild to severe in which one or more of the following can occur:[3]

- Hives/itching
- Tingling in the mouth
- Swelling in the tongue and throat
- Difficulty breathing
- Abdominal cramps
- Vomiting or diarrhea
- Eczema or rash
- Coughing or wheezing
- Dizziness
- Loss of consciousness or even death

Anaphylaxis

A severe allergic reaction that comes on suddenly and involves different systems of the body at the same time or causes difficulty breathing, swelling of the throat

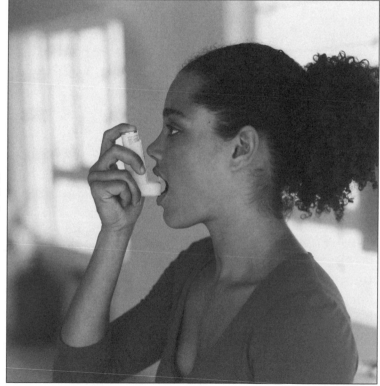

Food allergic reactions can also be more than a wheeze.

and tongue, or sudden drop in blood pressure is known as anaphylaxis.[4] It is important to note that there is no clear indicator of whether an allergic reaction will result in anaphylaxis. People can suddenly develop anaphylaxis from eating a food even if they have eaten the same food several times prior with little or no reaction. If not treated right away, anaphylaxis can be life threatening. According to Food Allergy Research & Education, although most symptoms of anaphylaxis occur within minutes of eating the offending food, symptoms of anaphylaxis can sometimes appear hours after eating the offending food. This is known as a biphasic anaphylactic reaction, and about 25 percent of patients who reported having anaphylactic attacks experienced a biphasic anaphylactic attack.[5] Although it is uncommon, it does occur and it is important to note that if the epinephrine is administered too late while an allergic reaction is occurring, the reaction may not be able to be stopped and can result in death. If you feel that you or someone you know is experiencing symptoms of anaphylaxis, do not hesitate to use an epinephrine auto-injector, which is the only proven medication to stop a severe or life-threatening allergic reaction, and call 9-1-1 immediately.

Epinephrine Auto-injectors

If you are not familiar with how epinephrine auto-injectors work, or have questions on how to properly administer the medication yourself, make sure to ask your allergist. There are several auto-injectors out in the market now, but you are probably most familiar with the name brands Adrenaclick, EpiPen, and Auvi-Q. If you go to any of these manufacturers' websites, there are instructions on how to administer the auto-injector properly. Sometimes they may even offer special manufacturer discounts or coupons that waive your copay fee, which you will be able to find on the website. Remember that each auto-injector device is different and may work a bit differently, so you will want to become familiar with the auto-injector that works best for you. Be sure to let your allergist know which auto-injector you find the best to work with or if you have a preference.

Even though the auto-injectors may work in a different manner, you must always remember to administer the epinephrine in the outer thigh. Once administered, the auto-injector usually has to stay in place for a few seconds to deliver the proper dose of medication. Be sure to go over the directions carefully when you speak with your allergist as well as when you pick up the medication. One difference between the auto-injectors is that the Auvi-Q auto-injector gives verbal directions. This may be a comfort to you if you do have to use the auto-injector while in the middle of an allergic reaction. It would also be helpful to anyone else who may find that you are having an allergic reaction and has to react quickly in an emergency situation. Oftentimes, when you do pick up your medication, there

Auto-injectors: Things to Keep in Mind

1. Always carry two auto-injectors with you at all times. This is very important in case something happens to the first auto-injector or if you find yourself needing a second dose before the ambulance arrives.

2. Auto-injectors are sensitive to temperatures. They usually need to be stored at room temperature. Never keep an auto-injector in the refrigerator. Never keep an auto-injector in the car.

3. If the solution of the auto-injector is discolored or contains particles, then make sure to replace it because the medication has gone bad. If there is any doubt whether there is discoloration, you may be able to take the auto-injector to your local pharmacist for her opinion, but be sure to replace the auto-injector anyway. You do not want to be in a situation where you need the epinephrine, and the medication is not effective. This is putting your life at risk.

4. Always be sure to check the expiration dates and be sure to obtain new medication if your current auto-injector has expired.

5. Be sure to dispose of your auto-injector properly. You can ask your pharmacist or allergist about proper disposal if you have any questions.

will be a trainer auto-injector included, which is just like the actual auto-injector except it does not contain a needle or medication. It can be a good way of practicing how to administer the epinephrine so you can become familiar with it. You can also feel free to contact the manufacturers directly, and they may be able to send more trainers if need be.[6] Additionally, with the assistance or supervision of your parents or guardians, some people use their expired auto-injectors to inject an orange to be continuously familiar with how to administer this life-saving medication.

If you have experienced anaphylaxis or feel that you have experienced symptoms of an allergic reaction, contact your allergist or doctor right away to go over the symptoms and get a thorough exam. In order to officially diagnose a food allergy, allergists take down your medical history and may perform a skin prick test.

During the skin prick test a very small amount of liquid protein is placed on the arms or back and then your skin is pricked with a small needle. Generally, after about fifteen minutes or so, if you test positive to a food allergy, a small bump will appear at the prick site as well as a slight rash. The bump will look much like a mosquito bite and will become very itchy. The size of the bump will be measured, and your allergist will go over all of the results with you to determine an action plan.[7]

In addition to the skin prick test, your allergist may also do a blood test to determine how many IgE antibodies to certain food proteins you have in your blood. However, even though the blood test may indicate high levels of antibodies, it is not a true indicator of whether you will suffer an allergic reaction to a particular food. In other words, even if antibodies are present, it does not necessarily mean that your immune system will react to these antibodies. The converse is also true. As mentioned previously, food allergic reactions can be non-IgE related and would therefore not show up in a blood test. In some instances, you could present with high levels of IgE to certain food proteins in your blood, but if these food proteins were altered by being processed or cooked, or even during the actual act of your body digesting the food itself, you may not ever experience an allergic reaction to these foods at all,[8] which brings us to the topic of oral allergy syndrome.

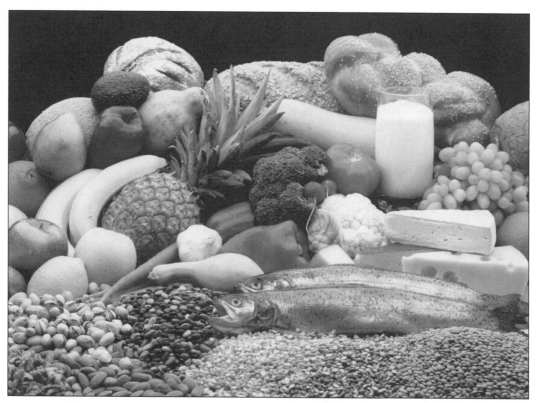

Although a majority of food allergic reactions come from the top eight foods, any food can cause an allergic reaction.

Oral Allergy Syndrome

Oral allergy syndrome is an allergic reaction to certain raw fruits and vegetables and is generally seen in people who suffer from hay fever. In hay fever, an allergic response is created by the immune system reacting to certain pollens that can be found in grasses, weeds, or trees. In oral allergy syndrome, the immune system confuses the proteins found in certain raw fruits and vegetables with those that are found in grasses, weeds, or tree pollen. This confusion by the immune system is known as *cross-reactivity*. Generally, if you or someone you know has experienced seasonal allergies or hay fever from grasses, then you may react to bananas or melons. If you suffer from seasonal allergies or hay fever from weeds or tree pollen, then you may find yourself reacting to pitted fruits such as cherries, peaches, plums, and so on.[9]

If you or someone you know suffers from oral allergy syndrome, the most common symptom that will manifest itself while the person is eating raw fruits or vegetables is an itchy, tingly sensation in the mouth, lips, and throat. Swelling of the mouth, lips, and throat may also occur. If someone is extremely sensitive, even touching raw fruits and/or vegetables can cause itchiness or a rash on the skin. Although it has occurred in certain individuals, very rarely does oral allergy syndrome result in anaphylaxis. This may be, in part, because simply by cooking the raw fruits or vegetables, the heat changes the makeup of the protein, which allows for just enough change that eating the food will not result in an allergic reaction.[10] With that being said, if you feel that this has happened to you, then you should talk to your doctor or make an appointment with an allergist to discuss your symptoms.

Never, ever, try to self-diagnose. Not only could self-diagnosis be dangerous if you suffer from multiple food allergies that could result in anaphylaxis, but you may be cutting food out of your diet for no reason if you feel that you have an

Cross-Contamination/Cross-Contact

Do not confuse cross-reactivity with cross-contamination or cross-contact. Cross-contamination is when proteins from one food are accidentally mixed with proteins from another food. People with food allergies need to be very careful about cross-contamination, especially when having meals prepared for them. An example of cross-contamination would be using the same cooking utensil to stir a cheese sauce, then wiping it clean, and using it to stir a noncheese item that was going to be served to the person who has a milk allergy.[d]

> **Other Conditions Associated with Food Allergies**
>
> The Kids with Food Allergies Foundation reports that if someone has a food allergy, she or he may be more likely to also suffer from asthma, eczema, eosinophilic esophagitis, or exercise-induced anaphylaxis.[e]

allergy and it has not been confirmed by a doctor or a board-certified allergist. Remember that there is no known cure for food allergies, and strict avoidance of the food is the best course of action you can take, along with carrying an auto-injector of epinephrine, which is the only form of treatment during a severe or life-threatening allergic reaction.

Food Allergies versus Food Intolerance

The misuse of the term *allergy* can cause confusion among the general population and may be why there is so much uncertainty or ignorance when it comes to fully understanding food allergies and how serious food allergic reactions can be. This is especially evident when some terms, such as *food allergy* and *food intolerance*, are used interchangeably, and they should not be, as they are two separate terms. Dr. David Stukus, board-certified in allergy/immunology and assistant professor of pediatrics, Nationwide Children's Hospital and The Ohio State University in Columbus, Ohio, differentiates the two by explaining that food intolerances are

Desensitization

Although there is no known cure for food allergies, there are studies being done to help with desensitization of an allergic reaction. Desensitization is a method that is sometimes used to allow people to tolerate greater amounts of an allergen before they suffer a reaction. This is always done by an allergist; never attempt this alone. "The Sublingual Immunotherapy for Peanut Allergy: A Randomized Double-Blind, Placebo-Controlled Multicenter Trial" conducted by Wesley Burks, MD, and David M. Fleischer, MD, showed promising results in children being desensitized to peanut.[f]

not IgE or immune reactions to a specific food. Symptoms are generally not as severe or immediate as with food allergies, and almost always involve some type of gastrointestinal symptom, such as feeling bloated, gassiness, heartburn, or changes to bowel habits. Intolerances may come and go over time, may only occur with a specific type of food preparation (may be fine with yogurt but cannot drink a glass of milk) or be related to amount ingested. There are no tests available to accurately diagnose a food intolerance and many people have to avoid a food for a period of time to determine if their symptoms go away, and then return when they eat that food again.[11]

As mentioned earlier, IgE stands for immunoglobulin E, which is an antibody found in the blood. When someone has an IgE-related allergic reaction, the IgE antibodies attach themselves to the protein of an allergen, which in turn triggers a response by the body's mast cells causing inflammation and an allergic reaction.[12] Basically, the important thing to remember is that food allergies involve the immune system, whereas having a food intolerance does not. Many people confuse these terms. A great example of this confusion is in the terms *milk allergy*, *dairy allergy*, or *lactose intolerance*. As mentioned, if someone is suffering from a milk allergy and milk is consumed by that person, the person's immune system will be affected and will cause an allergic reaction. So what exactly does having a dairy allergy mean? Well, here is where you will need to be careful about using terms correctly. *Dairy* refers to any product that contains milk. Proclaiming "I am allergic to dairy" or "I have a dairy allergy" may cause confusion for those who do not deal with a milk allergy directly and who may be reading ingredient labels for you since the labeling laws in the United States do not require "dairy" to be listed, but would instead list "milk" as an ingredient that may cause an allergic reaction. We will discuss ingredient labeling in the United States in greater detail later in the book since reading ingredients can be challenging for anyone, not just for those who are not used to dealing with food allergies. Additionally, someone who is not familiar with food allergies could mistake other products for dairy products when in fact they are not. One such product is eggs, as they are often stocked close to the dairy section in most grocery stores and supermarkets. A person who is allergic to milk would not necessarily also be allergic to egg and need to cut out egg from his or her diet.[13]

Gluten

Another widely misused and misunderstood term is *gluten*. There is a difference between *gluten intolerance/sensitivity*, *wheat allergy*, and *celiac disease*. They are most definitely not one and the same. Gluten is a protein that is found in wheat, barley, and rye, and there are many people who have self-diagnosed a gluten al-

> ## ! Did You Know?
>
> ● Do you know what Drew Brees (Super Bowl–winning quarterback of the New Orleans Saints), Elisabeth Hasselbeck (television personality), and Jennifer Esposito (actress, baker, author, entrepreneur) all have in common? They all eat gluten-free diets.[9]

lergy who may actually have a sensitivity to gluten or other food sensitivities or allergies that they are not aware of. This has caused confusion among the general population and may have caused certain individuals to eliminate foods unnecessarily from their diet. As mentioned previously, any food can cause an intolerance or sensitivity, including gluten, and it almost always involves the gastrointestinal system.

Celiac Disease

As you are now aware, an allergy invokes an immune system response. If someone suffers from a wheat allergy, the immune system overreacts to wheat, causing the typical symptoms of a food allergic reaction that has the potential to be life threatening. Celiac disease, on the other hand, is something else entirely as it is an autoimmune condition. Dr. David Stukus defines celiac disease as neither an allergy nor an intolerance, but is an autoimmune condition where the body will attack itself but only in the presence of gluten, which is found in wheat, barley, and rye. When

Jennifer Esposito

Jennifer Esposito suffers from celiac disease and is very active in the celiac community where she advocates for good, clean food. She opened Jennifer's Way Bakery, a completely gluten-free bakery, in New York City. In addition to her bakery, Jennifer also wrote *Jennifer's Way: My Journey with Celiac Disease—What Doctors Don't Tell You and How You Can Learn to Live Again*, a very good book for anyone dealing with dietary restrictions.

Gluten Free in the Supermarkets

Most supermarkets now have a gluten-free section with foods ranging from pastas and breads to sweets and baked goods.

people with celiac disease eat gluten, their body damages their own intestines, and can also affect skin, nervous system, and other organs as well. Symptoms can include upset stomach, bloating, diarrhea, or progress to skin rash, headaches, or fatigue. There are blood tests to help detect the autoimmune response to gluten, but using a scope/camera to take a biopsy of the intestine is the best way to diagnose celiac. The good news is that once celiac is properly diagnosed, most people do really well as long as they avoid eating anything with gluten.[14]

As Dr. Stukus mentions, celiac disease is an autoimmune disease, which means that it can affect many systems of the body. Additionally, since the disease begins by damaging a person's intestines, if left untreated or unchecked, it can cause problems with the way a person's body absorbs nutrients from any food, not just food containing gluten.[15]

Do Not Self-Diagnose

Again, if you notice that when you eat gluten or something containing wheat or gluten you do not seem to feel right, do not self-diagnose. Mention your symptoms to your doctor or allergist and have your doctor or allergist assess you from there. Many people who suffer from celiac disease go undiagnosed for quite some time, while people who may have no allergies or sensitivities drastically change their diet for no reason at all. Do not be one of these people. A good rule of

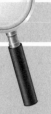

Remember the Differences

Food allergy = an unusual response to food caused by the body's *immune system*

Food intolerance = an unusual response to food caused by the body's *digestive system*

Celiac disease = an autoimmune disorder

thumb is if you feel a difference in your body from eating certain foods, begin to take notice. Do you get an upset stomach? Do you get a feeling of fullness in your throat? Does your tongue feel different? If you do feel a difference in your body when you eat certain foods, does it happen with certain kinds of food or when food is prepared a certain way? Start taking notice and keep a food journal. Any

It Happened to Me:
A Note from the Author Regarding Self-Diagnosis

I was twenty-one when I was diagnosed with having multiple life-threatening food allergies, but I began exhibiting signs of reactions to certain foods when I was a teenager. I remember my first allergic reaction to peanut butter very clearly. I was a freshman in college and had come home for the weekend. It was about 9:40 p.m. and I was hungry for a little snack. I decided that a peanut butter sandwich would be a good choice. I had eaten peanut butter my whole life, but for some reason when I was at college I did not eat it as frequently as I used to.

I went ahead and made the sandwich, but as soon as my tongue touched the sandwich it began to tingle and to burn. As I took a bite I realized that my mouth was feeling weird. My whole throat felt very funny, and it was becoming hard to swallow. I immediately did what any normal person would do in such a situation—I panicked and ran into my parents' bedroom. I could talk and still breathe even though my mouth and throat felt like they were slightly swollen. I was very lucky in that the reaction did not turn into anaphylaxis and subsided on its own after several hours. I then decided I must have an allergy to peanuts and stayed away from peanut products from that point forward without ever discussing it further with my parents or with a doctor.

This was a *huge* mistake. Since I had never encountered food allergies before, I did not understand what having food allergies really meant and I certainly had no idea about cross-contamination. I continued to have small reactions for years because I was ill-informed and self-diagnosed. Through the years, my reactions continued to get worse in nature, and now I am anaphylactic to peanuts as well as other foods. It was not until I ended up in the hospital due to an anaphylactic attack that I finally received my food allergy diagnosis, which changed my life forever.

time you eat a food and notice something different with the way you feel, write it down. By writing everything in a food journal, you can perceive if there are any patterns or similarities in the foods that seem to make you feel a little off. Not only will it help you, but it will also help your doctor or allergist in diagnosing whether you have a true food allergy, a food intolerance, or something else entirely like celiac disease.

As mentioned previously, food allergies and reactions related to food allergies are different for everyone who has them. Several people could be diagnosed with the same allergy, but one person may experience hives, one may have a fullness in the throat, one may have gastrointestinal problems, and yet another could suffer from anaphylaxis. It is best to discuss any symptoms with your doctor or allergist, and he or she can create an individualized plan for you on how to live a fulfilling life with food allergies.

Although being a teenager suffering from food allergies, food intolerances, or celiac disease can be difficult, it is doable. With a little bit of extra effort or adjustments to accommodate your condition, there is no reason why you cannot lead a fulfilling life. However, whether you have a medical condition or not, there is one universal truth that you will deal with as a teenager: All teenagers have to grow up and become adults. All teenagers are trying to find their way, to adjust to their roles in the world, and to start advocating on their own behalf. As with anything, some people have an easier time with this adjustment than others, but as a person who suffers from food allergies you will be able to practice these skills sooner rather than later because your life may depend on it. In the next chapter we will explore learning how to advocate for yourself and take on more responsibilities.

2

THE ART OF CALM-MUNICATING: BECOMING A SELF-ADVOCATE

O ne main thing that you need to remember is that being diagnosed with food allergies is *not* something you should be ashamed of and having food allergies is not a choice. No one would choose to have a swollen throat, a tongue that rises to the roof of his mouth, the air slowly leaving his lungs, all the while itching and breaking out into hives. According to the Centers for Disease Control and Prevention (CDC), children who are younger than three years old, or have a family history of allergy and asthma, have a greater likelihood of developing food allergies.[1] However, the fact of the matter is, any child or adult can be at risk for food allergies at any time, and studies have shown that allergies are on the rise in the United States and other developed parts of the world. The Food Allergy Research & Education website references another study done by the CDC that shows that from the year 1997 through the year 2011, food allergies rose in children under the age of eighteen by 50 percent.[2] Another startling conclusion from these studies is that the age groups that are at the highest risk for fatal reactions are teenagers and young adults. Please do not be frightened by that statement; rather, look at it as a wakeup call and work on trying to change this. Again, allergies are not something to be ashamed of and cannot be helped. The same holds true if you suffer from celiac disease. Look at these conditions as any other trait that a person has. Should you be ashamed that you are not the tallest person in your grade? Should you be ashamed that math comes easy to you? Should you be ashamed that you are a two-sport athlete and are equally talented in both sports? Absolutely not! It can get hectic and be a lot to take in, but now think back to a time when things were simpler. Take a deep breath and smell the tissue paper roses.

You read that right, tissue paper roses, like the ones you probably made in preschool or kindergarten. Do you remember what it was like being that age?

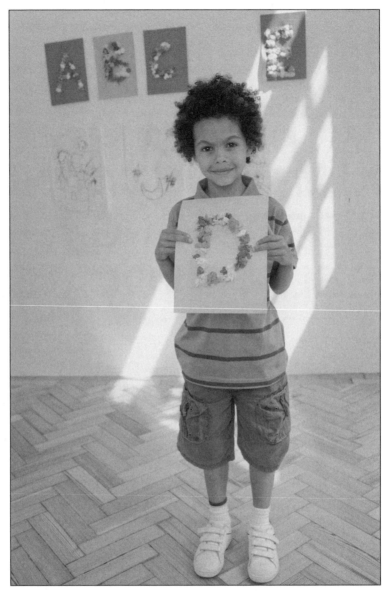

Remember when you were younger, and stop to smell the tissue paper roses.

Among other things, do you remember the importance of learning "please" and "thank you"? These words were most likely prompted with "What do you say?" and "How do you ask?" From the perspective of a preschooler or kindergartener, these questions might seem redundant and even lead to frustration. However, there really is an important lesson here that we sometimes forget as we get older. The simple question of "How do you ask?" is in and of itself a great question! We are taught at a very young age how to ask for things that we want or need in the proper way. Why, then, does this emphasis on learning how to ask for things stop as we get older? One reason may be that asking questions is perceived as annoying or needy. Rather than speak up for ourselves, some of us would rather suffer in silence. Additionally, no one wants to be thought of as being obnoxious and too outspoken for asking a lot of questions. However, when you are a person who has food allergies, asking questions can make the difference between having a good time and being safe and risking an allergic reaction, which at times could be life threatening. Asking questions and learning to advocate for yourself is an important aspect of learning how to live a fulfilling life with food allergies. The trick is learning how to ask such questions and what I would like to call the art of "calm-munication."

The *Merriam-Webster Online Dictionary* defines communication as "an act or instance of transmitting or a process by which information is exchanged between individuals through a common system of symbols, signs, or behavior." Now that you have the definition of communication in your head, let's think about communicating in terms of food allergies. You need to exchange vital information about the nature of your condition, and if you are talking about food allergies, there is the possibility of a life-threatening reaction. You may think that you have a good handle on managing your allergies, and if the time comes, you will tell people all about them. But no matter how great you are at managing your condition or whether you have a plan on how to communicate your dietary needs, sometimes things happen that are out of your control. Maybe you were waiting to find the right time to tell people that you have allergies, or maybe you were starting to talk about it and became frustrated because you could not seem to fit it in the conversation. Trying to deal with your food allergies and a busy lifestyle could be enough to make you want to scream or never even attempt to try to explain your needs. Please remember that even though there are things that are beyond your control, the one thing you always have control over is how you handle yourself in a situation; hence the term *calm-munication*. You hold the power to educate other people about your allergies and advise them on what they can do to help you during an allergic reaction or how to prevent illness. No matter what is going on around you, you need to convey the seriousness of your dietary needs and the steps a person needs to take in order to keep you safe. When someone gets upset or angry, what would you typically say to that person? That's right. You would tell her or him to calm down. It is very difficult to argue with someone or poke fun at someone who is making valid statements in a rational manner. Calm-municating and being able to advocate for yourself may sound difficult, but you can do it. After all, it has already been programmed into you from when you were younger.

Think back again to when you were younger. Now think of the riding-a-bike analogy. You were probably preschool or kindergarten age when you first learned how to ride a tricycle, and after a bit of practice, you were probably ready to try the big two-wheel bike with training wheels. Once you got the hang of the two-wheel bike and felt more comfortable, it was time to take the training wheels off.

Do you remember how that felt? You were probably excited to be able to try this out on your own, but still nervous about pedaling, and even worse, what if you fell? Your parent/guardian/grandparent, whoever taught you how to ride this bike, was going to be right behind you—and then you took a quick peek over your shoulder and realized that you were on your own! This probably startled you, caused you to swerve to the side, and then the unthinkable happened . . . you fell off the bike! Realizing that you actually had been pedaling and maneuvering the big two-wheel bike on your own, you most likely brushed the dirt off and got right back on, eager to try again. With a little bit of patience and practice, you

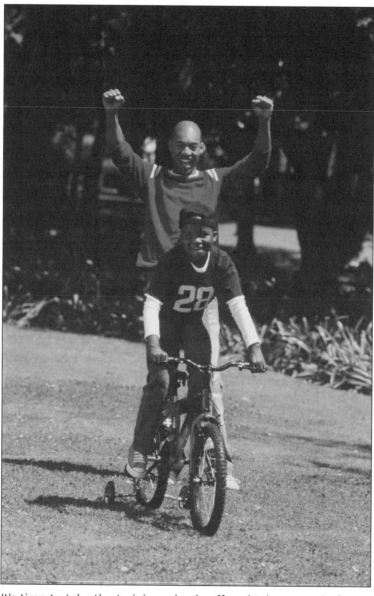

It's time to take the training wheels off and take control of your health.

became really good at pedaling. You did it! You learned how to ride a bike, a skill that you will most likely never forget.

Think of calm-municating and advocating your needs as like learning how to ride a bike. When you started riding a tricycle, you didn't have to worry about too much since you were low to the ground and there were not too many risks involved. When you were ready, you moved on to the two-wheel bike with training wheels, but eventually the training wheels had to come off and you had to pedal on your own. As you get older, you are given more responsibilities and are in more situations where you will need to learn the tools to keep yourself safe and healthy. Your family will always be there to support you, but as you get older, you may not see each other as often. Your mother or father may not be able to cook every meal for you. Just remember that you can do this! The other thing you must remember is that even the most vigilant of people make mistakes. Unfortunately, mistakes can and will happen, but if you have communicated your needs to others and expressed what to do in an emergency situation, then more often than not, everything will turn out fine. Still nervous about learning how to calm-municate? There is no need to worry. As mentioned before, you already possess all of the skills. You just have to tap into yourself and follow the steps.

Take Your Condition Seriously

The first step to calm-municating is to take your condition seriously. Food allergies are definitely annoying and can cramp your style during certain activities, but the symptoms should not be brushed off, particularly if you suffer from life-threatening food allergies. If you do not take your food allergies seriously, it will be hard for others to do so. People will need to know what happens to you during a reaction and what they should do in case of an emergency. Don't be one of those people who says, "It's no big deal; I just break out into hives." Although breaking out into hives is not always a precursor to anaphylaxis, it's still a serious symptom of an allergic reaction and should not be taken lightly.

Taking symptoms of a food allergic reaction lightly may be why many people think all allergy symptoms are just sneezing and itchy, watery eyes. The way food allergies are portrayed in the entertainment industry could also be a contributing factor to minimizing the seriousness of a reaction. For instance, stand-up comedians have used allergic reactions and those suffering from food allergies as punch lines in their comedic routines. The jokes are centered on the stigma that all people who have food allergies are frail and socially awkward. This could not be further from the truth. However, the more that those who have food allergies are silent about the seriousness of food allergies, the more misconceptions are allowed to fester and create misunderstanding.

In addition to being the brunt of the joke in a stand-up act, food allergy reactions are depicted as comedic in a number of movies and television episodes. These comedic scenes typically show the main character developing swelling and puffiness in the face, tongue, and throat, which renders her incapable of communicating effectively. Instead of addressing this as a serious medical problem, these scenes show the main character being laughed at because others cannot understand her. Miraculously, hours later, the puffiness and swelling have subsided and the main character is able to go about her business unscathed.

An example of one such movie is *Hitch*, starring Will Smith and Eva Mendes. Will Smith's character is attending a cooking class with Eva Mendes's character when he eats a food that causes an allergic reaction. His face begins to swell and gets puffy. Instead of calling 9-1-1 and using epinephrine, both characters run to a local pharmacy looking for a bottle of antihistamine. Will Smith's character downs the bottle of antihistamine and is taken back to the apartment of Eva Mendes's character, where he sleeps off the allergic reaction. When he wakes up the following day, all is right with the world. This scene is used in the movie as comedic relief and to allow a connection between the two characters wherein they discover they are developing feelings for each other. This is a recipe for a romantic comedy; however, this is not real life and certainly minimizes the seriousness of food allergies and what to do in an emergency situation if a food allergic reaction occurs.

In other movies or television episodes, food allergies may be depicted in a more serious tone, but the character who is experiencing the reaction never seems to have epinephrine on hand and, again, simply downs a bottle of what would appear to

Benadryl

Dr. George Rieveschl, who had a doctorate in chemistry, was an assistant professor researching muscle-relaxing drugs at the University of Cincinnati in the early 1940s when he realized the powerful potential of the antihistamine compound, which he later named Benadryl, then being tested as a muscle relaxer. With this new discovery, Dr. Rieveschl also noted that specific receptors in capillaries can be affected by different compounds. Antihistamines work to stop the histamine chemical from damaging capillaries in the blood, which then stops the blood plasma leakage that causes the inflammation associated with an allergic reaction.[a]

be a liquid antihistamine to stop the attack. Not only is this not funny, but it also inaccurately portrays how to treat an allergic reaction. If someone is experiencing an allergic reaction, especially an allergic reaction that turns into an anaphylactic attack, antihistamines will not do anything to stop the attack. As mentioned before, epinephrine is the only medication that can be used to stop a serious reaction. Because the seriousness of food allergic reactions is downplayed in this way, many people who do not deal with food allergies on a regular basis do not realize the severity and range of symptoms that can occur when someone is having an allergic reaction to food. This is why it is so important for those who do have food allergies to take their food allergies seriously and not minimize the symptoms of a reaction. In addition to not minimizing your symptoms of a particular reaction, part of taking your allergies seriously is to always have your medication with you.

Carrying around antihistamines like Benadryl or Alavert along with epinephrine can seem cumbersome. However, here are a few questions for you:

1. Would you run a marathon before running a 5K?
2. Would you go up against a 250-pound lineman with no pads?
3. Would you learn Spanish for your French Literature test?

Chances are you would answer (d) None of the above.

So why would you not carry your potentially life-saving medication? This is really a no-brainer. Just remember the phrase "Don't be scared to be prepared." Repeat it in your head as often as necessary.

If you are planning on going off to college, you will always need to carry around your dorm room key card. This card allows you access to your dorm and other campus facilities and serves as a campus debit card, allowing you to make purchases at the dining hall, bookstore, and so on. Basically, this card needs to be carried with you at all times. By keeping your medication with you now, you will be one step ahead in getting used to carrying something around in college. Plus, carrying your medication around is not only smart; it also reinforces the seriousness of your allergies.

> "I prefer to call my bag of EpiPens and Benadryl a satchel. Indiana Jones has one."
> —Spencer[b]

Be Open about Your Allergies and Your Reactions

Now that you are taking your allergies seriously, the next step is to be open about them and what happens to you during an allergic reaction, making sure to divulge enough information depending on the person. Although allergies are on the rise, not every person you encounter will know what to do if a reaction occurs or how to prevent a reaction. Many people who do not live with food allergies or who are not directly affected by food allergies do not grasp the seriousness of what happens during an allergic reaction, nor do they grasp the concept and reality of cross-contamination. For example, if you are peanut and tree nut allergic and someone eating a milk chocolate candy bar offers you some, that is cross-contamination. Although the ingredients themselves do not contain nuts, the candy was more than likely manufactured in a facility that also manufactures nut products. To someone with a severe allergy to peanut and tree nuts, even the most miniscule amount that could have ended up in the bar of milk chocolate candy would cause an allergic reaction resulting in anaphylaxis.

So, what do you do in this situation? Again, depending on the person and that person's relationship to you, the answer varies. If this person is someone with whom you do not interact on a regular basis and was just being polite offering you a portion, then a good response might be, "No thank you. I appreciate it, but I have food allergies." Done! Plain and simple. You are not putting yourself in a risky situation at this point because you are not ingesting any allergen. Nothing more needs to be said. Of course, if this individual asks you about your food allergies, then by all means educate him or her on food allergies to your heart's content. Never shy away from an opportunity to educate others and raise awareness. This person may need to help someone else with food allergies along the way, and you are just doing your due diligence in paying it forward.

However, what if this individual is more than just someone you see from time to time, but you still wouldn't consider her a close friend? You may frequent the same social events and run in the same friend circles, but for whatever reason she is still a fringe friend. In this case, it would be beneficial to talk about your allergies. If you are at the same events and with the same people a great deal of the time, it would be in your best interest to let the person know what's going on in case a reaction occurs. She may be wondering why you don't eat when you are at these events. You could begin the conversation with something like, "Hi, nice to see you again. In case you thought it was odd that I never eat when we see each other, I wanted to let you know that I have food allergies. I am allergic to [tell the individual the foods you are allergic to] and if I eat these foods I get an allergic reaction." It would be beneficial for you to discuss what happens during an allergic reaction and where you keep your epinephrine auto-injector. Always answer any follow-up questions she may have and, depending on your comfort level, even show her how to administer epinephrine in case a reaction was to occur.

If this individual is a good friend, then you should feel comfortable telling her your complete medical history, everything about your allergies, what happens to you during a reaction, who to contact if a reaction occurs, how to administer the epinephrine, and so on.

> ## When Should Your EpiPen Be Replaced?
>
> ● Even if the expiration date on the EpiPen shows it has not expired, if the solution is discolored or seems to have particles in it, the EpiPen needs to be replaced.[c]

The key to being open yet selective about the information you give depending on the individual is an important aspect of dealing with your food allergies on your own. Being selective about the information you give is especially important if you are ordering food at a restaurant. You have to convey to the waitstaff that you have food allergies to such and such a food and wonder if you can order anything off of the menu. You must do this in a matter of minutes and chances are you may not ever see each other again, but in this moment, you are putting your trust in that server's hands. You need to tell him or her about your allergies, and ask about the ingredients in certain dishes, but you do not need to go into your complete medical history. (Please see chapter 8 regarding ordering your food or dining in for more tips on how to handle yourself in a restaurant.)

Now that you are open about your allergies and talking about your needs, the next thing you need to remember is not to be offended if you find yourself repeating your needs to some people over and over again.

> "The more times you do it even if you are shy, the more confident you will be."—Alex[d]

Don't Take Offense

You take your allergies seriously and you thought that the people in your life were also taking your allergies seriously—until your friend brings a bag of trail mix to your house with every kind of nut you are allergic to. You begin to feel the anger rise up inside you and start to take over, followed by the urge to cry or lash out because how could your friend be so inconsiderate as to bring nuts into your own home? Before you get too upset, you need to remember that more than likely your friend did not do this on purpose. Yes, it was a slight lapse in judgment, but not because your friend doesn't care or take your allergies seriously. For you, allergies are something that you have to think about almost every time you eat something, and if you are one of those people who has an anaphylactic reaction, it's a life-and-death matter. You may think about it all the time. For teens not living with allergies, it is not an issue that they have to deal with on a constant basis; they may simply not remember your allergy. This is where calm-municating comes in.

Instead of freaking out on the person and getting upset, calmly remind him about your allergies and that you would prefer that he not eat the nuts around you. If this person is a true friend, he will probably feel terrible for putting you in an uncomfortable situation and not eat the nuts in your own home. You will now be able to move on with your day. Great, crisis averted. But what happens if something like this occurs when you are not on your own turf, so to speak?

If you are out somewhere or at a party and someone begins eating the trail mix with every nut you are allergic to, what do you do then? Again, kindly remind everyone about your allergy and what your reaction will be. Most of the time people will respond by putting the offending food away, but sometimes you will

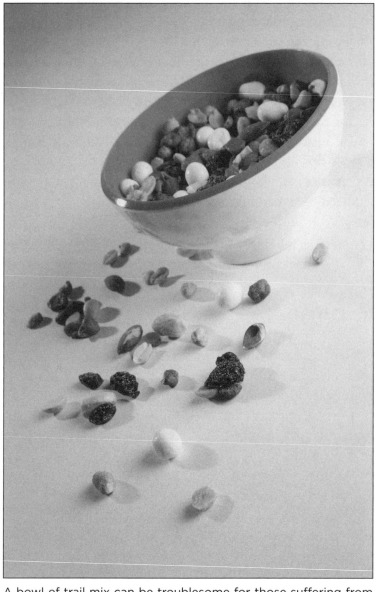

A bowl of trail mix can be troublesome for those suffering from peanut or tree nut allergy.

have to remove yourself from the situation. What if the individual who brought the trail mix is diabetic and that was the only snack she could eat? It would not be fair to ask her to stop eating the snack because that person's health would then be at risk. You simply need to remove yourself from the situation.

Sometimes you will need to remove yourself from the situation because people will continue to eat what they want without taking your allergies into account. Even with reminders and trying to educate people about food allergies, some people still do not understand or comprehend the seriousness of an allergic reaction. They do not understand symptoms of anaphylaxis and that having an allergic reaction is not simply breaking out into hives. Hopefully this does not happen too often, but it can happen—even among your family members. How to deal with family and friends will be discussed in greater length in the next few chapters, but in terms of calm-municating with family, friends, and others, the important thing to remember is to never be afraid to remind them of your allergies and your needs. It can get annoying and frustrating to remind people again and again, but when it comes to your health and safety, it's a small aggravation that is worth the trouble. It is very important to stay open about your allergies, and it is also important to remember to be open to repeating yourself and your needs. This will happen, so "don't be scared to be prepared."

Be Honest with Yourself

The last step in the art of calm-municating is learning to accept your feelings. If you can be honest with yourself about how you are feeling with regard to your condition, it will be a lot easier communicating your needs to another person and you will be taken seriously. For instance, to the friend who brought over the trail mix to your home, be honest with yourself. Would you be a little fearful you might have a reaction? Yes, maybe you would. Would you be a little hurt that your friend could have eaten any food and decided to bring the one food you could have an anaphylactic attack to? Yes, you might. Would you feel a little twinge of jealousy that your friend can eat whatever he wants without having to worry? Yes, probably. Guess what? It's OK. It is more than OK to have these feelings. It's perfectly understandable to have these feelings. Accept them and maybe even share your feelings so your friend can see where you are coming from. Then move on. Do not dwell on these feelings. Again, if this person is a friend, he did not forget your allergy on purpose. You have to accept that although your friend cares about you, it honestly might have slipped his mind due to other obligations going on in his own life. By the same token, if this were to occur at a party, you need to accept that in certain situations you may have to simply walk away.

We live in a world where allergens are around us all of the time. No matter how much you try to avoid the offending foods, chances are that you will end up

It Happened to Me:
A Note from the Author Regarding Calm-munication

Learning how to calm-municate can be tricky at first, but it is so helpful and important to learn. It can be used in any aspect of your life and may even be important when dealing with other medical professionals besides your allergist when it comes to your health.

In addition to being allergic to certain foods, I also have allergies to several medications. One of these medications is commonly used as an anesthetic. I was due to have a root canal (fun, I know), and upon scheduling my appointment, I verified my allergy and asked if I could have an alternative anesthetic that had been tested by my allergist and was approved for me to use. The office agreed that it would not be a problem. When the office called to confirm my appointment, I reminded them of my allergy and asked if the anesthetic I could have would be available. I was again assured that this was all set and not a problem.

However, when I appeared at the office for the appointment and stated for a third time that the anesthetic that I was to be given was not the one I was allergic to, the endodontist looked annoyed and said that he was unsure if he had the other anesthetic in stock in the office. To say that I was absolutely infuriated is an understatement as I had given them ample time to get the correct anesthetic and now I was going to have to come back if they did not have the right one. I kept my cool and calm-municated to the endodontist that he might want to check in the office or with someone else on his staff because I had called twice to confirm the correct anesthetic was available for me for this appointment and was assured that it was.

Luckily, the crisis was averted and they were able to find the anesthetic that I could have, but the endodontist did not put away the one I was allergic to. Before he did anything I asked him to put it away and just leave the one I could use on the dental tray. Both anesthetics looked like the little sample perfume bottles, and they were the same color so it would have been very easy to mistakenly use the wrong anesthetic. Instead of simply putting the anesthetic that I was allergic to away, the endodontist argued with me and was offended that I would even question his knowledge, letting me know that "I have been doing this a long time and I know which is which." Using my calm-munication skills, I simply replied that while I believed him, it would make me feel better and it would be in his best interest to put the anesthetic I was allergic to away. That way, he would not risk the chance of giving me a reaction.

After this incident the office manager advised me that the office would be going over their allergy policies in more detail and apologized profusely. While this was simultaneously a scary and aggravating experience, it may not have resulted in a positive outcome if I had not used calm-munication. Again, it is very difficult to argue with someone if she or he is calm and making valid points.

being around those foods at one time or another. It would be wonderful if people could cater to your needs, but the world doesn't work like that nor should it, which is why you will need to take an active role in calm-municating your needs when necessary. *The* world may not be looking out for you, but your immediate sphere of people who create *your* world will. If you keep practicing the art of calm-municating with those around you, the population of *your* world will grow larger and larger and allow you to live a fulfilling life.

Let's review. The steps to effectively calm-municate are

1. Take your condition and dietary needs seriously. For those who suffer from food allergies, always carry your medications with you.
2. Be open about your needs. Do not be afraid to share information, but not everyone needs to know your complete medical history.
3. Repeat your needs and what to do in an emergency situation, and then don't be afraid to repeat it again, or again and again. Sometimes you may need to walk away.
4. Accept your feelings so that you can identify your needs and calmly discuss what your needs are in relation to your allergies or celiac disease. Keep practicing calm-munication skills and build up a world that will support you.

FAMILY: FROM HARSHEST CRITICS TO BIGGEST CHEERLEADERS

Dealing with food allergies creates challenges not just for those living with food allergies, but also for the people who interact with those who are affected, namely, family members. The notion of "family" can be different for everyone. Some people come from small families where they are only around immediate family members. Some people come from large families where the immediate

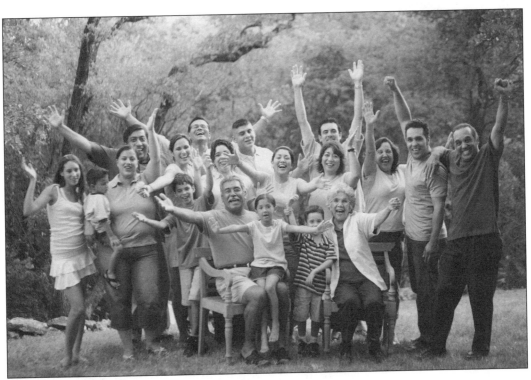

Family should be there for you as your biggest supporters.

family members may include five siblings. Other people may have a small immediate family but have a large extended family with whom they interact on a frequent basis. Whoever your family members may be, one universal rule remains the same: each family member needs to know about your allergies. Additionally, those family members who interact with you on a frequent basis should know what to do if an emergency situation occurs.

> "Growing up with a sister that has many allergies is hard, but seeing what she has to endure everyday has changed my perspective."—Gracien L.[a]

For those of you who were diagnosed as infants or early on in your childhood, your immediate family is most likely well aware of your allergies and how to live with them. You most likely are a well-oiled machine and have a food allergy routine down pat. Whether it be joining local support groups, cooking all of your meals, or making sure to travel with all of your medication, your family has been there for you. From a young age, you had parents, grandparents, or other caretakers navigating the "new normal" by making sure to keep you safe and helping to prevent allergic reactions. You may honestly have been so young that you grew up not knowing any other way, but here is where it can get a little tricky and is a normal outcome of growing up and getting older. Whether you suffer from food allergies or not, part of growing up is learning to become self-sufficient, self-aware, and a self-advocate. Since you grew up with your family doing most of the heavy lifting, so to speak, the responsibilities that come with being a teenager, especially a teenager with food allergies, can, at times, seem overwhelming.

As a teenager, taking an active role when it comes to living with your food allergies may seem too much to handle on your own or something that you do not think you have to worry about until you get even older. You might be thinking that it is something that you can handle if you decide to go off to college or move out on your own. You know what to do and will deal with it at a later time. The truth is, to do anything well takes practice, including managing your food allergies. Hopefully you have not had to suffer an allergic reaction in quite some time. If you have not had a reaction in a while, do you remember what to do if a reaction were to occur? You hear your parents, grandparents, or caretakers explaining to other people, including other family members, about your allergies and how to manage them, but have you explained your allergies to these people yourself? Have you been the one to show others how to administer epinephrine if a reaction were to occur? Do you remember how to administer epinephrine to yourself if the situation were to arise? If you answered no to any of these questions, it's OK. Whether you have never really thought about any of these questions or are

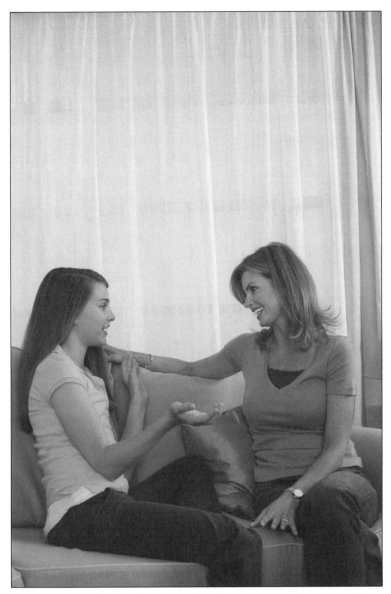

Do not be afraid to talk to your family about everything troubling you regarding your allergies.

a bit embarrassed to admit to your diligent family that you are unsure about what to do, it does not matter. What matters is that you are now taking the steps to re-familiarize yourself with how to handle your food allergies. Talk to your family to discuss your concerns.

It may also be a good idea to make an appointment with your allergist to have a consultation about what you should be doing in terms of allergy management now that you are older. Remember, doctors are not just there to give you medications and physical checkups. They are a great resource in dealing with the management of your allergies as well. It is never too late to take an active interest in your health, and there is no better time to start than right now. With that being said, what if you are always an active participant when it comes to dealing with your food allergies, but feel as though certain people in your family are the ones who are not allowing you to take on a more active role in your food allergy management?

It is completely understandable if your parents, grandparents, or caretakers seem a little too overprotective when it comes to your food allergies. Put yourself in their shoes for a moment. They were most likely the ones who witnessed your first food allergic reaction and felt helpless and frightened that this could possibly be happening. In some cases, they could have been the ones who caused the reaction by eating an offending food and giving you a kiss on the cheek, which resulted in a welt, a full-on anaphylactic attack, and a trip to the emergency room. While you have grown up with a food allergy routine, they were the ones, through trial and error, who had to put the routine into place. For your entire life, they will always want to keep you safe and take care of you.

> "Let go and give me a chance to show I am responsible."—Alex[b]

The ongoing struggle for a little independence from family is something that all teenagers have to deal with. However, this struggle can be even tougher when you are a teenager with food allergies because it can be frightening for your parents, grandparents, or caretakers to give you this independence, even though they know that this is something that needs to happen. Up until this moment, they have been the ones advocating for you and making sure that you are safe when it comes to your food allergies. They have also been the ones to teach you how to manage your allergies, and now is your time to shine. Put their fears at ease by showing them that you have listened to everything that they have taught you and that you are ready and willing to put their words into practice. Maybe this means attending a food allergy support group that they have been members of since you were diagnosed. Start asking to carry your own allergy medications with you. When you go to your next allergist appointment, be the one who asks the questions or talks to the allergist more than the family member who goes with you. Offer to go grocery shopping with your parent, grandparent, or caretaker to pick out your own safe foods and even offer to help with the cooking. If you go out to eat at a restaurant, be the one who takes the initiative to discuss your allergies with the manager, waitstaff, and/or chef and then allow members of your family who happen to be with you to add any additional comments. By actively initiating conversations you are showing your family not only that you want more responsibility, but that you are capable of more responsibility. Always remember the art of calm-municating as mentioned in chapter 2 and apply it to everyone you can, including your family. Wishes and concerns are always better received if they are spoken in a calm and cool manner rather than with screaming and shouting as you run off to your room thinking no one understands where you are coming from. While communication is key to any relationship and mutual understanding, there will at times be those family members who will simply never understand. What do you do in this situation?

As food allergy sufferers, we have all been there; the holiday party where it is inevitable that the topic of food allergies will come up, feelings will get hurt, and we ask ourselves why we allow this to happen every year. It is sort of a rite of passage as a member of the food allergy community, and for those of you who were diagnosed later on in childhood or in your teens, this can be even more difficult. For family who do not interact with you on a regular basis and who are not familiar with food allergies, there are lots of questions and judgments. They may perceive food allergies as not real or that you are being fussy. When you pull out your safe food labeled with your name from the fridge, they may make snarky comments or even call you a hypochondriac instead of listening to what is really going on. It is more important than ever that you try to calm yourself and use the art of calm-munication. Educate these family members as much as you can by explaining about food allergies, what happens during an allergic reaction, and the issue of cross-contamination. It may take the course of several holidays in order for certain family members to understand or simply stop asking questions. It is not uncommon for certain members of the family, year after year, to ask such questions as

- "So, are you still allergic to the same foods?"
- "Have you tried any new foods since the last time we saw you?"
- "Did you bring your own food again?"
- "That must be really frustrating. What can you eat?"
- "Does it bother you watching us eat such good food that you can't have?"

While these questions may be fine if answered once or twice, getting them year after year even after you provide the same answers can seem like an endless cycle of frustration and anxiety when attending holiday parties. Additionally, it causes added stress for you and your immediate family during a time when you should be celebrating. Understanding may not happen overnight for those family or family friends who seem to have a hard time acknowledging your food allergies and grasping just what it means to have food allergies and everything that entails. It may take numerous times for everything to click, and unfortunately, in some cases, understanding may never happen.

If understanding never happens, there are a few ways you can handle this. First, you can continue to try to educate them, hoping that one of these times it might sink in. Second, you can try to switch the focus of conversation on them.

If you are directing questions to them, it will be difficult for them to focus on you. If they do switch the focus back to you, there is a third option and that is being straightforward, stating that you "agree to disagree." Never be disrespectful, but you can simply say in a nice way that food allergies are part of your life, including bringing and eating your own food, and even if they do not agree or have comments, they need to talk about something else because the focus should be on the holiday and not on your food allergies. However, before you enact this third option, it would be a better idea to tell someone in your immediate family or family who live in your household about the issue and they can jump in for you. Sometimes when dealing with extended family members or family friends, it may be best for your immediate family to take the lead. If the extended family members and family friends are spoken to by everyone else attending the holiday party, they may think twice about negatively commenting about your food allergies. Additionally, if these certain invitees are causing you too much anxiety and grief, your parents, grandparents, or caretakers may decide to decline next year's invitation until these certain people can become more understanding or simply accept that it is a way of life for you and something they should not comment on. Although the decision to decline an invitation lies with your parents, grandparents, or caretakers, always discuss how you are feeling and how other people are making you feel when it comes to dealing with your food allergies. Additionally, the host of the party may not invite these family members or family friends the following year if it seems to be causing too much conflict or anxiety. It is so important to create an environment where you feel safe, including feeling safe both physically and emotionally.

While immediate family members such as your parents, grandparents, or caretakers are usually your first line of support when it comes to food allergies, in some rare instances, they may be the very ones who need your help to fully understand what you are going through. In certain cases, especially if you have been diagnosed later on, your immediate family members may not fully grasp what it means to live with food allergies. Instead of asking the same questions over and over again, certain family members may act differently toward you. This difference is not rooted in maliciousness. Rather, it is your family trying to not make you feel like you are missing out on something. However, in doing so, they create more of an awkward situation, which can be just as bad as the incessant questions.

For instance, say you are at a holiday party and you just walk into the room. Everyone is surrounding the appetizer table and filling their dishes. Some relatives may even be grazing at the table while simultaneously putting food onto their plates. When you arrive, everyone stops talking and stares at you wide-eyed with a guilty look on their faces. You proceed to greet everybody and hear some of your relatives say not to kiss them on the cheek because they had a food you are allergic to. They may go on to say that the food was not that good anyway and not to worry that you cannot eat it; you were definitely not missing out. This statement may be followed up with additional negative comments about the food at the party or about the way a certain food was made. You may even notice some relatives making additional comments that they think will make you feel better, such as

- "I *wish* I had food allergies, then I wouldn't be overweight. I would be forced to eat well and then I could look like you."
- "It would be amazing if I had food allergies, then I could learn how to cook like you."
- "There are too many food choices out there and if I had food allergies, then the choices would be made for me. Life would be so much easier."
- "If I had food allergies I would probably save *so* much money on going out to eat and getting coffee every morning. You're really lucky."

Although your family members may think that they are making you feel better by trying to identify with you, these comments can be just as insensitive as outright mean comments about your food allergies. Foods that a person consumes are a choice. Learning how to cook would be a choice. Spending money on certain social activities like going out to eat is a choice, just as getting coffee instead of making it at home is a choice. Food allergies are *not* a choice. No one would wish to have food allergies on purpose. Additionally, negative comments about foods that are probably delicious and took a lot of time and effort to make are silly and unnecessary. Although you have food allergies, you can still appreciate that foods you are allergic to may in fact be quite delicious, and it is okay for those family members and you to express that the food looks good.

If this sounds like a familiar situation for you, then just realize that these family members are trying to keep your best interest at heart. Their comments and awkwardness happen because they do not want to hurt your feelings or make you feel any different than anyone else in the family. In addressing these relatives, you can just be completely honest and let them know that you are aware that they are trying to make you feel comfortable, but it is perfectly okay for them to enjoy foods that you may not be able to eat, as long as they are keeping you safe by washing their hands and not kissing you on the cheek after they have had something you are allergic to. You can also let them know that you appreciate them trying to make you feel included, but you have your own safe foods that are delicious and perfect for you. Putting down the foods that someone else spent the time to make or provide for the party is wrong as well. As long as your relatives are mindful of your allergies and are not putting you at an unnecessary risk of an allergic reaction, then they should view your eating habits the same as everyone else's. For instance, maybe one of your aunts prefers anything with chocolate while another aunt prefers a more fruity-tasting dessert. When asked what they would like for a dessert, the first aunt chooses the double-dutch chocolate cake with buttercream frosting while the second aunt chooses to have a slice of lemon merengue pie. No further questions would be asked of them regarding their preferences for dessert. In fact, if this is a big party, then there are probably numerous desserts to choose from. More than likely no one would be asking each other why a certain dessert was chosen over another. No one would be watching intently with wide eyes every time a bite was taken. Everyone would be enjoying his or her own respective dessert. You may also find some relatives who would choose to forgo the dessert completely and have a coffee instead, and most likely no one would think twice about it. The conversation would simply move right along, and it would be assumed that the relative who is choosing to have a cup of coffee is too full from the large meal that was just eaten. Dealing with your food allergies should be quite the same way. You may be eating different things, but you do not have to be treated differently. Your food allergies do not have to be the focus of everyone's attention or conversation as long as everyone is mindful of your allergies and not putting you at risk for an allergic reaction.

Another issue that you may run into when dealing with family is that they may understand that you can have an anaphylactic attack from certain foods like nuts, but they may not fully comprehend the idea of cross-contamination or the fact that you can have an allergic reaction that does not result in anaphylaxis, but can still cause difficulty swallowing, itchiness, and anxiety, which makes it harder for you because people may not believe that you are truly having an allergic reaction.

If you have ever suffered an allergic reaction as a result of food someone cooked for you, you may have a hard time trusting that person to cook for you again. This is especially difficult if it was a family member who cooked the food that caused the reaction. You may experience great anxiety because you do not want to come right out and say that you do not trust that parent, grandparent, or caretaker to cook for you because he or she raised you, and you do not want to hurt his or her feelings. For instance, let's say you are anaphylactic to nuts and have a bad reaction to other foods such as egg, and your mother is cooking dinner and decides to make something new. She went to the store and meticulously read every ingredient label searching for the ingredients that would cause you to have an allergic reaction, including egg. It certainly smells delicious and you ask

"At any moment of any day, my life can depend upon a half-inch needle containing .3 milligrams of adrenaline. One person's careless mistake can send my life into a whirling fight for survival."—Katie L.[c]

her what she is making. She explains that she is trying a new recipe, but it is allergy safe and she labored in the grocery store aisle to read all the ingredients so it would be something that you can have. She wants to cook something different for you instead of just the same safe meals. You may ask just to see the box so you can read the ingredients yourself, and as soon as the question leaves your lips and reaches your mother's ears, you can see the hurt behind her eyes. She may come back at you defensively asking how dare you not trust her, especially since she spent an extra hour reading ingredient labels just for you to make sure you have a nice dinner and something different. She would never cause you an allergic reaction. You are her child, and it is her job to keep you safe. She would never intentionally do something to hurt you so no need to check the ingredients. How would you deal with this scenario if it happened to you?

While it can be difficult to challenge your mother, or any family member for that matter, especially if she is trying to do something nice for you, it is really about your comfort level. You should always feel safe and comfortable in your own home, and it is certainly not unreasonable to ask to double-check the ingredients on a box for a meal that is being prepared. The key point in the preceding scenario is the fact that a mother tries to do what she thinks is best for her child. If this scenario happened to you, you would need to discuss your concerns with your mother indicating that although she is your mother and you know that she took a long time at the store to read the ingredients to ensure they are safe, since your last bad allergic reaction, you have an uneasiness about trying any new foods, no matter what. Although she is your mother, it would make you feel better just looking over the ingredients yourself to confirm their safety. You are sure that this uneasiness will pass as you become more comfortable eating food cooked from different recipes, but you just need her to be patient with you until it passes. If you talk about your anxiety or what you need to feel better in a calm manner, although your mother may not understand why you still have difficulty trusting her, she will hopefully do everything she can to put you at ease. Your trust issue is not a reflection on her but developed from a bad experience that you had, and you will need your mother's help to move forward so that you can get past the bad experience and be open to trying new recipes as long as you know they consist of all safe ingredients.

Another issue that may come up, especially if you come from a large extended family, involves someone cooking a safe meal for you while at the same time cooking a different meal for the rest of the family, which contaminates your safe meal. How would you handle this situation?

Say, for instance, your family is all on board about your food allergies and how to keep you safe. In fact, your family is generally good at cooking allergy-friendly meals for you. You and your immediate family always go over to your grandmother's house on Sundays for pasta with sauce and a variety of appetizers. You, your mom, and your dad always offer to bring a safe meal for you to make it easier on your grandmother because, after all, she is getting older and it's a lot of work to prepare so many different meals, but she will not hear of it. She is determined to cook for you so you can enjoy the same type of meal as the rest of the family and have the same experience. It would be an insult to her if you brought over your own food.

You arrive at your grandmother's house and can smell the sweet tomato sauce before even entering the kitchen. She must have been cooking the sauce at a simmer for hours. Excited to see you, she starts talking and you take a seat at the kitchen table. You notice that there are several pans on the stove—one pan is sauce for you and the other pan is sauce for the rest of the family. As you chat with your grandmother, you notice a big bowl with one or two roasted chestnuts sitting in front of you on the kitchen table. Your grandmother notices the fear and anxiety in your eyes and quickly rushes over to grab the bowl out of your way. Although you are not anaphylactic to chestnuts, your throat does swell a little among other symptoms of an allergic reaction. She apologizes for having them out, and since there's only one or two left, she goes into the next room to eat them so they will not cause a problem and comes back in the kitchen. She washes the bowl and washes her hands several times.

You settle back down into your conversation as she continues to stir the sauce, and that's when another mistake happens. Not only did she forget to change spoons between the sauce for you and the sauce for the rest of the family, but she also tasted the sauce for you and the sauce for your family with the same spoon. Not only is your sauce cross-contaminated now, but remember the chestnuts? Your grandmother diligently cleaned the bowl and washed her hands, but you don't remember seeing her brush her teeth so now your safe sauce may have chestnut protein in it along with other ingredients from the other pan of sauce that you are allergic to. You feel terrible that this happened, excuse yourself quickly, and see your father in the next room. You tell your father what happened and that you can't eat the sauce now and ask how you can say this nicely to your grandmother. Instead of understanding and providing you with a solution, your father lets out a sigh. He then asks you if you can just eat a little because you're not anaphylactic and your grandmother worked really hard to make a special meal for you. He points out that she would be devastated if you didn't eat what she cooked and asks if you could just be a little uncomfortable so that you don't hurt her feelings. Additionally, neither you nor your parents brought any safe foods for you to eat, so you would be stuck without any food and you most likely were going to be at your grandmother's for several hours. Has this situation ever happened to you? What would you do in this situation?

There are a lot of things going on in the preceding scenario, and unfortunately, situations like this happen. Although it's not an easy situation to deal with, it can and must be dealt with. You certainly do not want to hurt anyone's feelings, but your health and safety are in danger and that is never OK. In order to address the situation, you would first need to address your father's response. Although your father would never intentionally hurt your feelings, that is exactly what happened in this scenario, and it seems as though he is choosing your grandmother's feelings over your own and over your health and safety. While it was not your father's intention to do this, this is in fact what is happening, and you would need to calmly bring this to his attention. Also, asking you to be uncomfortable for the sake of your grandmother's feelings downplays the seriousness of your allergies and allergic reactions, which is taking a few steps back in making the family allergy aware.

After your father is aware of what transpired, it's time to speak to your grandmother. She, of course, would be very upset because she tried so hard to make a good meal for you, but ultimately she did this out of love, which is what you have to remember. Because your grandmother loves you, she wants you to feel comfortable. Yes, she may be upset that she contaminated your safe food. Yes, she may be upset that she worked so hard on your meal that you now cannot eat. Yes, she may feel bad that you may have to eat something that is not like the rest of the family, but she will get past that. She loves you and wants you to be safe. Plus, the sauce can be eaten by other family members without a problem, so it will not go to waste.

Additionally, this scenario is a great example in showing that no matter where you go, even if it is the most trusted of places, you should always bring safe foods just in case. As mentioned earlier, mistakes can and do happen. It would be better to have your safe foods with you and not need them, than not to have anything to eat. It is so important to remember to always be truthful with family members about your food allergies and concerns you have about food that is being cooked for you. It is a big responsibility to cook for someone with food allergies, and whoever does take on this responsibility needs to be aware that if a mistake is made, then the person with the food allergy will not be able to eat the food that was prepared. This is something that comes with cooking for someone with a food allergy. It is a big responsibility but not an impossible one, and of course, it gets easier with practice each and every time. With that being said, there is another important aspect about dealing with family and your food allergies, and that is to show your appreciation for everything that your family has to go through to make you safe, such as in the following scenario.

You have been away at a summer camp for several weeks, and now it's time to return home. You get picked up by your parents and then start bringing all of your belongings into the house. As your mom is bringing your dirty laundry downstairs to be washed and your dad is pulling the car into the garage, you decide to get a quick snack and a drink from the fridge. You open the fridge and notice that there is an egg carton in there, which is strange because you are allergic to eggs and your family never buys them. You grab some water and then proceed to the cabinet, where you are shocked to see a jar of peanut butter on the top shelf and the jar is almost finished. You are allergic to peanuts and you thought that your family did not like these foods anymore because they never buy them.

When your mom comes up the stairs and sees your look of shock, she apologizes for having the foods in the house and quickly calls your dad to get rid of everything. Your dad quickly gathers the offending foods and takes them away, apologizing some more. You turn around confused, but your little brother is there to answer your questions. He tells you that he's sorry that they had these foods in the house, but since you were away, they could eat them in the house again. When you reply that you thought no one liked the foods, your brother laughs and shakes his head. He tells you that of course they still like the foods; they just eat them outside of the house and not around you because they want you to be comfortable and to keep you safe. The truth is, you never really thought about the things that your family may also have to give up or the fact that they, too, need to make concessions on a daily basis even though you are the one with the food allergies.

Whether your family forgoes a favorite snack you are allergic to, declines certain restaurant invitations, or spends hours cooking special meals, it is so important to let them know that you are aware of the many things they do for you and you appreciate it. Although family can be the source of disagreements and your harshest critics at times, ultimately they are always there to support you, to cheer you on, and to keep you safe. When your family is not around, you still need to surround yourself with people who can support you and with whom you can share your interests in a positive manner. These people are your friends, and the following chapter will explore friendships, especially friendships pertaining to keeping you safe with regard to your food allergies.

It Happened to Me:
A Note from the Author Regarding Family

Since I was diagnosed with multiple food allergies at the age of twenty-one, it was a steep learning curve for both me and my family. It seemed that just when we all were on the same page with regard to my allergies, something would happen to prove otherwise. However, by talking about all of my concerns and worries with my family, we learned together and got a good system going. After we discussed all of my concerns, my family has been nothing but supportive and I honestly would not be where I am today without them. So, as difficult and aggravating as it can be sometimes, be sure to talk about your feelings with your family.

FRIEND OR FRENEMY?

I n the last chapter, we discussed how important it is for family to be on board with you when it comes to your food allergies. It is equally important for your friends to be on board and understanding. If you think about it, in a given day you may spend just as much time, or maybe even more time, with your friends as with your family. Since a good friend should know you inside and out, she should be prepared to assist you in regard to handling your food allergies. With that being said, let us explore what it means to be a friend.

Take a look at the two pictures on the page. You may notice some similarities, such as both pictures have a group of friends sitting at a dinner or restaurant table. However, it is more important to note the differences in the pictures. Notice the expressions on the faces of the friends in the first picture versus the expressions on the faces of the "friends" in the second picture. In the first picture, the friends are

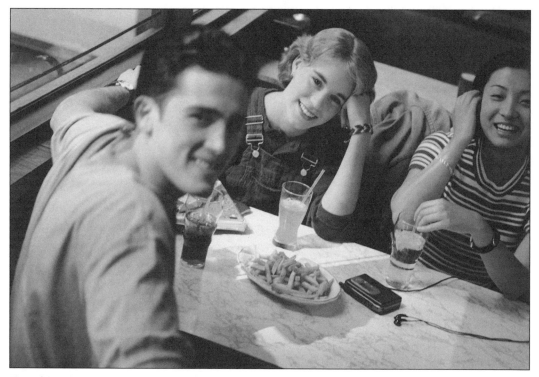

True friends are there to support you and lift you up.

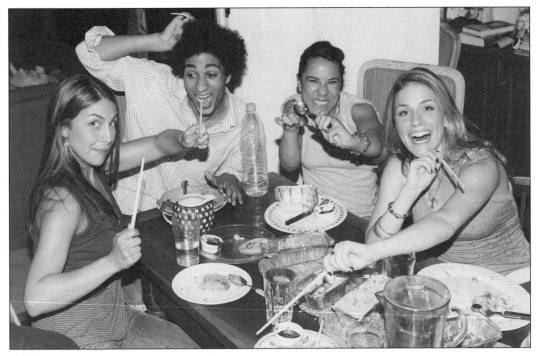

Frenemies—people who act like your friends, but do not have your best interest at heart.

sitting down to a meal with food in a clearly defined area. They have welcoming expressions, and if you are someone with food allergies, these look to be friends who understand what you are going through in regard to your allergies. In the second picture, the expressions of the friends, or "frenemies," look to be antagonizing and possibly malicious. In fact, it looks as if one of the girls in the picture is pretending to throw food in your direction. Sometimes there is a very fine line between joking around and being hurtful. However, when it comes to food allergies being hurtful, *hurtful* can mean causing both emotional harm and physical harm. Whether the girl would have in fact thrown the food does not matter. Clearly, these people in the second picture would not be taking your allergies seriously. The carelessness shown to your emotional and physical health does prove one thing: these people are not your friends.

> "Friends end up becoming a problem when they are having a negative influence on the person's life."—Lee[a]

Circle of Friends

As you enter different stages throughout your life, it is not uncommon to change your close circle of friends. If you are entering high school, you may even start to see this change occurring right now. If this does not sound like you, consider yourself lucky to have found a close group of friends you can continue to grow with. However, if this does describe you, then not to worry; it is completely normal on the road to growing up. If you have lost touch with some of your childhood friends, you may discover that years down the road you may become reacquainted. Whether you are still close with these friends or you seem to be drifting apart due to other interests, those experiences you had together when you were growing up will forever be a part of you, including these friends learning how to assist you with your food allergies.

When you were a child, your parents, grandparents, or caretakers most likely spoke with the neighborhood families and raised allergy awareness. In doing so, allergy awareness would transfer directly to your childhood and neighborhood friends. From a young age, your childhood friends probably knew what it meant to have food allergies, what foods you are allergic to, how to keep you safe by not eating those offending foods around you, and to get the help of a trusted adult at the first signs of an allergic reaction. You most likely never gave it a second thought at just how well-versed your young friend or friends were at dealing with your food allergies. You probably spent time outdoors, playing games, and simply being a kid, which is exactly what you should have been doing. Allergies were, and still are, a part of you, but when you were younger you were not solely focused on what your friends thought of you with regard to your food allergies; you were more concerned about the next activity and hanging out. Why, then, should this completely change as we get older? Granted, with age comes responsibility and more self-awareness, and with that, self-consciousness and concern about how we are perceived by others. These are all normal feelings as you enter your teenage years, and unfortunately, some adults still suffer from worrying about what other people think of them. Do not turn into one of these adults, and if you are experiencing these feelings, do not let these feelings last long. Be confident in who you are and everything that makes you, you, which includes embracing that allergies are a part of your life.

Good Friends

> "Never be so overly cautious that you won't go out with friends."—Spencer[b]

If someone is a good friend, then she or he will embrace everything about you. Good friends are always there to support you whether you are having a good day, a bad day, or any day in between. They are honest with you even when you sometimes do not want to hear it. They know you inside and out and help you to become the best self that you can be as you try to make sense of life together.

As you continue to branch out to other activities, sports, or clubs, your circle of friends will widen. Even though the people within your friend group may widen or change, the core of what being a friend is all about should never change. If people want to hang out with you because of how well you performed at a sport, because you got first place in a club competition, because you can assist them with their homework, or because of the amount of money you may have, these people are not your friends. If you continue to be true to yourself and who you are, you will attract people who value you as a person and as a friend. Additionally, if you are involved in extracurricular activities or sports, it is inevitable that friends are going to be made because of your shared common interests. From these common interests, experiences will occur, stories will be shared, trust will develop, and voilà! A new friendship has been born in which you will continually learn more about each other as the friendship develops.

An important aspect of friendship is to keep each other in check and balance. In doing so, you also have a vested interest in keeping each other safe because you care about each other's well-being, which includes your friend knowing about your allergies. Now here is an exercise for you to try. Put yourself in the place of your friend. What if he was the one who had the food allergies, and you were the one without them? You would want your friend to tell you everything that you needed to know about how to keep him safe with regard to food allergies. If you

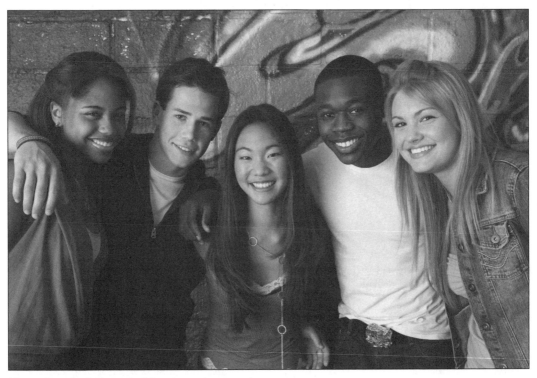

Never be afraid to gain friends and expand your crew.

were not familiar with food allergies, you would want to become familiar with them because you care about your friend and his well-being. You would not mind knowing which foods your friend is allergic to, and if he was highly sensitive, you probably would not mind foregoing a snack or meal that contained that allergen just so you could all have a good time and enjoy each other's company. You would want to know how to help your friend if an emergency situation occurred and you had to use his auto-injector.

Now, back to being you again. You most likely realize that not only is telling your friend about your food allergies and how to keep you safe necessary, but it is really not that big of a deal. It is nothing to be embarrassed about. In fact, if you have delayed telling your friends what they need to know, then there is no better time to start than right now. As you continue to get older, your trusted friends will not only be there to socialize with you, but they will become your biggest supporters, advocates, confidantes, and maybe even taste testers. When you go out to other social events, your friends should be there with you to make sure you are comfortable. Some may even go above and beyond that and help you form your own advocacy campaign or platform, which is exactly what happened with the founding of Nutties for a Change.

Nutties for a Change is an online forum complete with website and blog (nuttiesforachange.wix.com/nfac) that seeks to eliminate food allergy ignorance and also serves as a resource for those living with food allergies. It was created by Tiffani P., a thirteen-year-old food allergy sufferer, with the assistance and support of her best friend. Tiffani was tired of seeing the lack of understanding that other food allergic teenagers receive from their peers, so she decided to do something about it, especially since her own best friend supports her so much. Tiffani wants to drive home the fact that food allergy education and awareness are essential for anyone suffering from food allergies, but more so among teenagers suffering from food allergies. It is so important not to be self-conscious about your allergies because these insecurities can lead to closing yourself off from your friends and peers. Tiffani advises, "Wherever you are take a moment to educate your friends or peers about your allergies. If you don't share, they won't know. As inconvenient as it may seem, aware them. It's much more pleasurable to be informed of allergies, than to rush to an emergency room."[1]

As with anything, the more you address your needs and talk about your allergies and how to deal with them, the easier it will be each time you do it, and you will feel better off in the long run as well. Heidi S., a teen adviser with Food Allergy Research & Education (FARE) who is peanut and tree nut allergic, says that she discusses her food allergies with her friends quite often, and sometimes it seems that it may come up on a daily basis. Heidi says, "Usually whenever someone starts to eat something I can't identify, I ask them if it contains nuts. My friends also make an effort at parties and things to make sure there's food that's safe for me. And whenever I meet a friend's parents, it's usually 'Remember, Mom? She's the one I told you about who's allergic to peanuts!'"[2]

Food Allergies Are Not a Joke

Even though friends can be your biggest supporters, some of them can also make offhanded comments when it comes to your food allergies that serve to be funny, but may in fact be hurtful to you. This can happen, but know that more than likely if your friends are supportive of you on a daily basis and are usually your strongest advocates, they do not mean to hurt your feelings. Since you would discuss anything with your friends, make sure you let them know that these comments feel hurtful. If they are your good friends, they will not make such comments again and will feel bad about hurting your feelings.

With that being said, you may think some people are your friends, but when faced with certain social situations, they may not be truly supportive of you and go with the crowd, so to speak. Take it as a life lesson and cherish those friends who do support you on a daily basis through thick and thin. If you have experienced people wanting to be your friend because of what you can do for them or if they do not support you when faced with certain social situations, then recognize

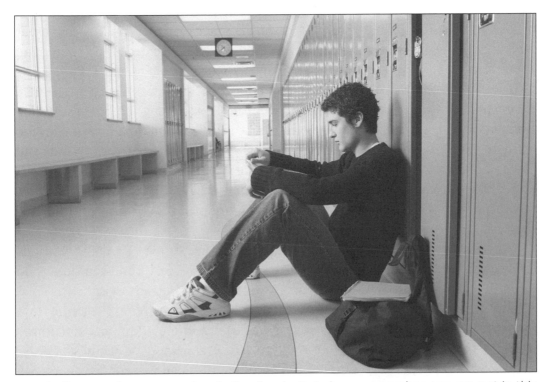

Hurt feelings can leave you sad or feeling lonely. But always remember: you are not in this alone!

"My friends at lunch ask if they can eat certain things in front of me. I usually say they can eat whatever they want as long as they wash their hands when they're done."—Michelle G.[c]

that these people are not your true friends. Additionally, if your so-called friends are always putting you down or poking fun at you, then they are not your true friends. Depending on the situation, the actions of these people could even be a form of bullying.

Bullying

Unfortunately, whether food allergic or not, some teenagers experience bullying. Bullying is defined as "unwanted, aggressive behavior involving a power imbalance that can either be real or perceived as real and occurs repeatedly. This aggressive behavior can occur by attacking someone verbally, physically, or excluding someone from a group on purpose."[3] Bullying should never be tolerated and

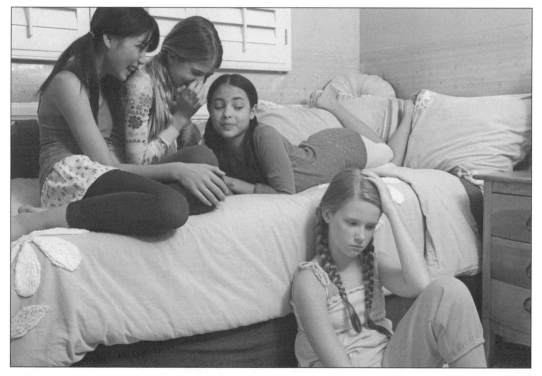

Bullying can come from anywhere. Be sure to address bullying as soon as it starts and tell a trusted adult.

can be emotionally and psychologically difficult for those who have been affected. However, being bullied as a result of food allergies not only can cause hurt feelings; it can cause a situation that is immediately life threatening.

According to FARE, about one-third of school-age kids with food allergies have reported being bullied at some point during their life as a direct result of having food allergies.[4] In my discussions with teenagers while writing this book, some reported that they have not been bullied at all, while others reported they have been bullied because of their allergies. Some of those who have experienced bullying reported that not only have they been bullied, but they have been directly bullied with the actual allergen itself. For those teenagers who were directly bullied with the allergen itself, the bullying ranged from peers pretending to eat the allergen and pretending to throw it in the way of the food allergic teenager, to actually touching the allergen and then leaving traces of the food on the food allergic teenager's lunch while laughing. All of the teenagers who were interviewed, whether they were bullied or not, reported that they believe food allergic bullying is a problem. Whether bullying is verbal alone or the actual allergen has been used to taunt and tease, there should be no tolerance for it and there are resources out there to help. Whether you are the one who is experiencing bullying or you have been a witness to bullying, the first thing that you need to do is to tell a trusted adult that it is occurring.

Additionally, according to FARE, about half of those who reported being affected by food allergy bullying never mentioned to their parents that they were being bullied.[5] It is understandable that you may be apprehensive about telling your parents, but you should always keep open communication with them about what is going on. If you feel that this is out of the question and you cannot talk to your parents, please talk to a trusted adult who can guide you on what to do. If you are the one experiencing the bullying, then oftentimes it may feel like you are alone, that there is no way the bullying can stop, that there is nothing anyone can do. This is definitely not true! There is always an answer, and there are always steps you can take to make a situation better. Unfortunately, bullying did not just come into existence; it is something that schools have needed to deal with for decades. If you are experiencing bullying or if you witness it, be aware that most schools have plans in place on how to handle bullying and have policies on

> "I have had isolated instances in which parents or kids either refuse to invite me to a party or make fun of my allergies. I just whisked it off as a fluke and carried on with my life. One person's opinion doesn't define you, so you should embrace who you are and carry on."—Jake H.[d]

the subject. By talking about bullying with your parents, a trusted adult, or your friends, you will not only be able to deal with the situation, but hopefully put a stop to it for good. Dr. David Stukus had this to say when it comes to food allergy bullying:

Bullying can affect every aspect of someone's life from school performance to engaging in extracurricular activities, and even sleep quality.

While it is sad that more and more children and teenagers are developing food allergies, this has made it a bit easier to deal with, as more people are now aware of the dangers. Unfortunately, there are still a lot of people out there who do not understand or believe in how severe food allergy reactions can become. There are several educational tools available through major organizations including Kids with Food Allergies, Food Allergy Home, and Food Allergy Research Education that can be downloaded or printed and shared with others.

Additional Resources Regarding Bullying

For additional resources regarding bullying, please check out the following:

1. www.stopbullying.gov. This website provides information regarding bullying from a number of U.S. government agencies. It addresses such issues as defining the different types of bullying, how to deal with bullying if it occurs, cyberbullying, and how to prevent bullying.

2. www.pacerteensagainstbullying.org/tab/about-us/. This is a great website geared specifically toward middle school and high school students about the topic of bullying, how to address it, and building a community that promotes safety and wellness.

3. The It's Not a Joke campaign created by FARE on its website (www.food allergy.org/its-not-a-joke?#.VMJKmS463LE).

4. Another great book in the It Happened to Me series—*Bullying: The Ultimate Teen Guide* by Mathangi Subramanian, EdD (Rowman & Littlefield, 2014).

It Happened to Me:
A Note from the Author Regarding Friends

When I was first diagnosed with food allergies, it was extremely difficult for me to get used to because the very foods that I had eaten a week before could now be potentially harmful and cause anaphylaxis. I was very lucky to have supportive friends who helped me navigate this new lifestyle. They were there for me to taste foods first when we ate out at restaurants and were willing to go to the same restaurant chain over and over again because it was where I felt comfortable eating. As we got older, they provided (and still provide) "Jess-safe" foods for me when I go over to their houses. When I was pregnant with my first child and put on bed rest, one of my friends cooked meals for me that could be frozen and heated as needed. I am so fortunate to have such good friends who support me for who I am. Always remember that friends should be there to lift you up and not to tear you down.

As much as possible—speak up! Anyone who is bullied is not alone, even though it may seem like it. Bullies take advantage of someone's perceived weakness, and use that to torment that person. Not only is having a food allergy not a weakness, but almost every classroom has someone with food allergies in it—so you're not alone![6]

When it comes to bullying, keep in mind that most people are not inherently bad. A lot of conflict can arise simply out of ignorance. Most bullies act out because they are missing out on something in their own life or are being bullied themselves in some other way. They need to feel a shift in power in order to feel better about themselves. Every person has their own ups and downs as well as their own insecurities that they must deal with. Always keep lines of communication open with your parents, trusted adults, and your friends. The good friendships that you have established can help in creating a safe and fun environment for you as you continue to experience the joys and struggles of growing up. These good friends will be by your side no matter what. They will be your allergy wingmen and women at social events like parties and in helping others understand your needs when it comes to your allergies.

PARTIES AND ATHLETICS

The topic of parties was mentioned briefly in earlier chapters when discussing holiday parties with family and friends. In this chapter the topic of parties and athletics will be discussed in greater depth as it pertains to friends and peers. Unfortunately, peer pressure can surface at any time and from many different people. Sometimes, peer pressure can even come from those closest to you without those friends realizing that they are putting you in an uncomfortable situation. When it comes to parties, the important thing to remember is that just because you have food allergies, it does not mean that you need to compromise having a good time. What it does mean is that you will need to be prepared and be responsible when it comes to making sure that you keep yourself safe. This means always carrying your medications with you and, at times, only eating and drinking food and drinks that you bring to the party yourself.

If you have had allergies your whole life, you are probably used to dealing with birthday parties. Your parents, grandparents, or caretakers were probably the ones to RSVP on your behalf when you were young, and speak to the party host about your allergies. Depending on the host's comfort level and allergy awareness, your immediate family would decide whether you would be able to eat at the party. If the party host was not comfortable preparing or was unable to provide safe foods for you, it would be no problem for your mom or dad to pack some safe foods. Now that you are older, you are going to be attending more friend parties on your own without having your immediate family there to assist you. You will have to decide on your own whether the foods are safe for you to eat. Depending on how severe your allergies to certain foods are, a general rule of thumb is to always eat before the party and to bring safe foods with you to eat while at the party. Remember, even the most diligent of your friends can get caught up in a conversation and not realize that they could have possibly contaminated a bowl of nachos by touching a food you are allergic to and then digging through the bowl to get the largest chip. Additionally, parties are much more than snacking on nachos, cake, and ice cream. They are about socializing with your friends and peers. Spark up a conversation or politely involve yourself in someone else's circle of conversation. Be engaging, but most importantly, just be yourself.

More than likely, if you are attending a party at a close friend's house, he and his parents are aware of your allergies. Maybe your friend's mom was sure to get pizza you are not allergic to from the local pizzeria. Maybe your friend's mom enjoys cooking and is friendly with your own mom and made sure she cooked something allergy friendly for you. If this describes you, then you are a lucky friend. Your friend and friend's family have given you every reason to feel comfortable eating around a group of people in this setting. Additionally, because you are surrounded by people who know you well, not only should they be aware of your allergies, but they should also know what to do if you have an allergic reaction. The same should hold true if you are attending a team or club dinner.

If you are part of a sports team or involved with a club at your school, chances are you will have to attend a team or club dinner at least once during the season. Oftentimes, these dinners are hosted at a fellow teammate's or club member's home. In this instance, you could speak to your parents, grandparents, or caretaker and ask to be the host if possible. That way, you can ensure that there will

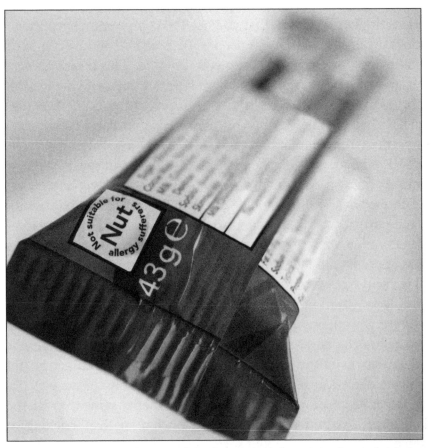

Nut protein bars are often a quick go-to snack for a lot of people, so be aware of what people are eating around you.

be an abundance of safe food you can enjoy since it will be in your own home. Even if your family is not able to host the dinner and it is at another teammate's or club member's house, these people should know enough about your allergies and what to do if you were to have an allergic reaction. Just think—if you are a quarterback of the football team, you have a center and an entire offensive line protecting you during a game. Your teammates are willing to put themselves out for you to protect you, and most assuredly they will want to protect you both on and off the field.

You got through the team or club dinner and everything turned out fine, but what happens at the end of the season and your team or club dinners are not in someone's home? What happens if these dinners are now at a restaurant or at a banquet hall? Well, more than likely your family will be attending this event with you, and you can talk it over with your coach, adviser, parents, grandparents, or caretakers. Check over the menu plans and see if accommodations can be made for you. In most instances, this should not be a problem and you could work with your coach and family members to make sure it is both a safe and enjoyable experience for you. Again, it is always a good idea to eat before you go out and also bring a few safe foods or snacks. This will ensure that in the off chance something happened to the special food request you made and you were not able to eat it, you have a backup, which is never a bad thing.

For the most part, those teenagers who are active in teams or clubs and who were interviewed as part of this book had a good relationship with their teams and coaches. They felt comfortable speaking with their teammates and coaches

> "I am on my school's volleyball and cross-country teams. When we have pasta parties the night before a game, I always mention my nut allergy and request nut free food."—Katie O.[a]

> "I am on the soccer team and the team knows about my food allergies. My coach and teammates are careful about the food that we have for snacks at games and at parties. A few of the other girls on my team also have food allergies so this has made it easier on me because more girls and their parents are aware of food allergies."—Zoe P.[b]

> "I have made sure that my coach is aware of my food allergy, how to use my EpiPen and where the EpiPen is located. I make sure that the team knows not to eat or bring nuts anywhere near me."—Kayla S.[c]

regarding their allergies and how to handle an emergency situation if it were to occur. However, after I spoke with these teenagers, it also became clear that there is not a universal approach on how to handle food allergies in the athletic world, and it is even more apparent that the seriousness of food allergies is really only understood when it is presented in terms of a peanut or nut allergy. Unfortunately, this is something that seems to be prevalent not only in the athletic world, but also among the general population. With that being said, it is so important to remember that *all* allergies should be taken seriously, and that, depending on the person, even if a food allergy is not part of the "top eight," it can still cause anaphylaxis and should be taken seriously. The following interview with Alex N. addresses a lot of these issues. Alex, a student-athlete who is a Teen Advisor for Food Allergy Research & Education (FARE) and who is anaphylactic to artificial dyes, preservatives, and sweeteners, had this to say:

I wanted to become a Teen Advisor for FARE because anaphylaxis to artificial food additives is not a topic that is normally discussed. I wanted to bring the voice of someone who does not have one of the "Big Eight" allergies to the table. I also wanted to get people talking about athletics and anaphylaxis. To the best of my knowledge, there are no resources for athletes affected by food allergies/anaphylaxis, and FARE has no outreach groups to educate the athletic community, such as coaches and athletic camp staff, about food allergies and anaphylaxis. My role as an advisor is to act upon FARE's mission statements of education and outreach by helping other people who have been diagnosed with food allergies/anaphylaxis and spreading awareness to the global community.

I am currently part of a USA Swimming Team and also swim for my high school team. I have discussed my anaphylaxis with my coaches. They are all aware of my anaphylactic reaction protocol and have been instructed on how to administer an EpiPen. Nearly every coach I've had has been comfortable with handling my anaphylaxis. At one point, however, I had a coach that was afraid of being sued by the aquatic center that employed him, and he required one of my parents to be at every practice and meet. He would not even learn my anaphylactic reaction protocol because he was afraid of the possibility of a lawsuit. This experience is what turned me into an advocate for athletes with food allergies/anaphylaxis.

I have experienced anaphylaxis on multiple occasions. I carry my EpiPen with me everywhere at all times, no matter how inconvenient it is. I use a small running pack to put my Benadryl, oral prednisone, and two epinephrine auto-injectors. I keep the pack in my backpack, swim bag, or pocket. I guess I will put it in my briefcase when I have a professional job. The medicine in epinephrine requires a temperature range of 59–86 degrees, so I do not leave it in a hot car, and keep it in a cooler at the beach. I keep it in my ski jacket when I ski, or do other outdoor winter sports. I have trained all of my friends, my friends' parents, and my relatives in the proper use of an EpiPen. My anaphylaxis has never stopped me from traveling. Over the years, I've found ways of dealing with my anaphylaxis on the road, and my family has been very supportive of me. My parents find hotels near restaurant chains that are safe for me, like Panera Bread or the hot bar at Whole Foods Market.

I've dealt with my food allergies at school by making sure all teaching staff are instructed on the proper administration of an epinephrine auto-injector and my anaphylactic reaction protocol, giving a duplicate set of my medication to the school nurse, and carrying my epinephrine auto-injector on me at all times. In respect to eating, the only way for me to have a meal is by bringing my own, so I've negotiated the use of a staff microwave and use it to heat up my lunch. The school will not provide a microwave in the general cafeteria, so I have to use a separate one in the staff office.[1]

When I spoke further with Alex, he brought up a good point regarding comfort levels when eating at events. Although you may have formed a comfort level eating at team or club events or parties with your good friends, you may not feel so comfortable when you attend a party at a place that you are not so familiar with or with other attendees you do not know very well. Alex went on to say that he is "just coming to the point where saying no to food at a party feels normal," and this situation may occur more and more frequently as you get older. Your circle of friends gets larger as you involve yourself in more activities or after-school jobs or internships. While you may know the host of the party and one or two other people, you may not be familiar with the other attendees. In some instances, you may not know the host all too well but were invited by other close friends of yours. Does this mean you should not attend this or any other social event because you do not know all of the other guests or hosts that well? Absolutely not! Just be prepared as you would when getting ready for any other type of event. Make sure you eat before you go to the party and bring food with you as well as all of your medications.

Most importantly, however, when it comes to going to a party where you do not know everyone or are not familiar with the party location, you will need to bring at least one trusted friend with you. If that trusted friend was not initially invited, make sure to ask the host if she would mind if your friend came along as well. It is important to have a trusted friend with you in case an allergic reaction occurs. As mentioned previously, not everyone in a room needs to be well versed in how to handle your food allergies. If the topic comes up or food is offered to you that you cannot have, it would be logical and beneficial to inform this person or group of people about your allergies. If they have follow-up questions, then be sure to answer them. If they seem OK with you just passing on the food and they move on to the next conversation, then that is fine, too. As long as you have at least one trusted friend who knows what to do during an allergic reaction and is there to offer support for you, then you should be sure to have a good time. However, there may be times when your supportive friend, or friends, puts peer pressure on you without meaning to. How would you handle the following situation?

Say you were invited by a friend to a party at one of her friend's houses, someone you do not know too well. You decide to go because the friend who invited you has been your friend for quite some time. She is a person you feel safe and comfortable around, and you have been to parties with that person before. "This should be fine," you think to yourself and decide that you do not need to drive this time and you will go with your friend since you are not too familiar with the street the party is on.

You get to the party and hit it off with the host right away, which is not surprising since the host is a friend of your friend. You realize you have similar interests and you have a lot to talk about. Your friend sees other people she knows and asks if you would mind if she goes to talk to these other friends while the host is giving you a tour of the house. Of course you don't mind and proceed with the tour, meeting new friends and having a good time. When the host brings you back to where the party is, your senses perk up and your throat tightens. There is no mistaking that smell. The strong scent of salt and roasted peanuts fills your nostrils. Although you would have to consume the peanuts to become anaphylactic, you will get other symptoms if someone at the party eats them and touches your skin with a handshake or a kiss on the cheek. You politely excuse yourself from the host and search out your trusted friend, who seems to be hitting it off with the person you both have been crushing on since you were in the fifth grade. Watching from afar, it looks like the two are finally hitting it off and you hate to interrupt this moment, but you need your friend. You take your friend aside and instead of the reaction you were expecting, your friend asks if you could just give her a little more time because things were really starting to go well. Your friend tells you that the two of you will definitely leave, saying, "Just make sure you don't eat anything or touch anyone and you should be fine, right?"

Can you guess the key word in the last sentence of that previous paragraph? That's right; "should" is the key word. Never, under any circumstances, feel as though *should* is good enough. Saying you *should* be OK provides room for error and does not give the confidence that you *will* be OK. Although mistakes can and do happen, and sometimes they happen even when you are the most prepared, you want to make sure that you are always taking the necessary steps to feel safe and OK. The fact that you knew your friend was engaged in a potentially life-changing conversation with her crush and you still needed to interrupt because you did not feel safe means that you needed to address the situation right away.

Have you decided how you would handle the situation yet? As with anything, there are a few different ways you could go about it. First, of course, is taking your friend aside and letting her know exactly how you feel. You go on to say that you are afraid of an anaphylactic attack because of the peanuts and not knowing who has been in contact with them. It's making you very uncomfortable to be in this situation, and you really cannot stay at the party. If this is a good friend of yours and you are fearful of putting yourself in danger, she will absolutely leave the party. Maybe you can give the crush your friend's phone number and tell the person to give your friend a call. The other thing to point out is that if you are going to a place where there are a lot of unknowns, there is a chance that you might have to leave. You should be sure to either take your own car or have transportation available to you by calling a parent, older sibling, or another friend to pick you up. Backup plans are necessary for everyone, but when you have life-threatening food allergies, they are essential for your safety.

The other way you could handle the situation is by going to the host directly and informing him about your food allergies. A good host wants to ensure that everyone is safe and having fun. If you explain the severity of your allergies and kindly ask the host to remove the peanuts, more than likely your request will be granted. If for some reason, the host cannot accommodate you, then this is where a backup mode of transportation home would be essential. In most cases, you probably will not have any issues, but you do need to plan ahead just in case.

Another way you could completely avoid the issue of encountering snacks you may be anaphylactic to is by informing the host of your allergies ahead of time. If the host is a friend of your friend, then your friend can help begin the conversation. If your friend begins the conversation for you, the host will be aware of what snacks can be served without sending you into anaphylaxis, even if they are things that you still cannot eat because of cross-contamination. The host can also tell other guests not to bring snacks containing your allergens, so you can go into the party more confident that you will be safe. Be sure to eat before the party and bring additional safe foods for you to snack on. If you would like to go one step further, you could even offer to bring some snacks to the party. Whether it is store-bought snacks that you know you can eat without a problem or something you made yourself, bringing food to share is a good icebreaker and can prove that just because something is allergy safe does not mean that flavor or taste is sacrificed. Allergy-safe snacks can be enjoyed by everyone. The number of allergy-friendly bakeries is increasing all the time, and some bakeries may make special accommodations if asked.

Try Snacks from These Allergy-Friendly Companies

You can bring a dessert from Divvies (www.divvies.com), chocolate from Vermont Nut Free (www.vermontnutfree.com) or Pascha Chocolates (paschachocolate.com), or a snack from Enjoy Life Foods (enjoylifefoods.com/our_foods/), or try your hand at baking yourself with an allergy-friendly mix from Cherrybrook Kitchen (cherrybrookkitchen.com).

Another important factor to mention when discussing parties is the topic of underage drinking, especially in relation to food allergies. Plain and simple, underage drinking is illegal and illegal for good reason. In no way is this book trying to condone underage drinking, but the fact of the matter is, underage drinking does occur. According to the U.S. Department of Health and Human Services' *Surgeon General's Call to Action to Prevent and Reduce Underage Drinking*, alcohol is the most widely used and abused drug by American youth and is a major public health problem in America.[2] Additionally, the Office of Juvenile and Delinquency Prevention reported a startling statistic: people aged twelve to twenty years old drink 11 percent of all of the alcohol consumed in the United States. Out of those people, more than 90 percent of the alcohol that is consumed is in the form of binge drinking.[3] The National Institute on Alcohol Abuse and Alcoholism defines *binge drinking* as a pattern of drinking that brings a person's blood alcohol concentration to 0.08 percent or above. When discussing underage alcohol use among teenagers, the Surgeon General warns that underage drinking can affect the following:[4]

1. *Your actual brain*: Since the brain continues to develop as you enter young adulthood, if you engage in underage drinking on a regular basis, it can actually change the development and structure of your brain. Scary thought, isn't it?
2. *Your decision making*: As you may already be aware, consuming large amounts of alcohol can significantly impact thinking skills, allowing for poor decision making. Some poor decisions would be to drive a car while under the influence or to be a passenger in a car being driven by someone who is under the influence. You may also find yourself engaging in risky sexual behavior, which has a whole list of additional negative consequences including unwanted partners, sexually transmitted diseases, and unwanted pregnancy.

3. *Your behavior patterns*: If you are too focused on partying and under-age drinking, you may be falling behind in school and beginning to get a negative outlook on life in general. This negativity can lead to patterns of substance abuse with alcohol and other drugs and a path that you should not want to go down as it can cause damaging effects to all aspects of your life, including the possibility of legal issues.

4. *Your life*: Injuries due to underage drinking are a major cause of death among young people. Such injuries result from motor vehicle accidents, homicides, suicides, drowning, burns, falls, and so on.

The aforementioned is something that all teenagers should be aware of and concerned with when it comes to underage drinking. However, as a teenager with food allergies, you will need to be even more aware of the potential consequences of underage drinking since your life is at risk if you have an allergic reaction, not just by getting behind the wheel of a car or in a car with someone who is under the influence. Just think about it—if you are at a party where everyone is drinking and people are not thinking as clearly and logically as they should, do you really think that your allergies are going to be the first thing they're concerned with? Unless you are directly affected by food allergies, being aware of allergies and cross-contamination is a lot to take on and to remember. If the people you are with are under the influence of alcohol, it may not be their intention to put you at risk for an allergic reaction, but they may honestly forget about preparing safe food, not having the offending food at the party, or reminding other partygoers that you have an allergy and maybe refrain from eating an offending food. Additionally, if the host of the party or the party attendees cannot remember you have allergies, do you think they will know what to do if you begin to exhibit signs of an allergic reaction? More than likely, they will not. With that being said, you also cannot hold other people responsible for maintaining your safety when it comes to your food allergies.

Although it is extremely important to have supportive friends and even a whole network to support you, it is ultimately your responsibility to keep yourself safe. What do you think would happen if you became under the influence at a party or drank more than just a few sips? What if your crush is the one to offer you some food that may or may not contain your allergy? You may be so under the influence that you cannot think clearly, and you may decide to take the risk of eating the food so as not to make a big deal out of your allergies. Or you may be so intoxicated that all rational thinking goes out the window, and the chance of an allergic reaction may not even cross your mind. However, if you were to have an allergic reaction from eating that food, it would be a big deal. More than likely, your crush would feel terrible for having been the one to provide the unsafe food.

There's another factor that you need to consider if the thought of drinking crosses your mind, and that is you may actually be allergic to your alcoholic beverage. You may not be aware of an allergy to alcohol until you actually ingest the alcohol, and, for obvious reasons, you will not want to find this out at a party where everyone is under the influence. For instance, if you have a wheat allergy, you are probably aware that most beers are derived from wheat and grains and, therefore, drinking beer is not a wise decision for you. However, even if you do not have a wheat allergy, you could have an allergy to baker's or brewer's yeast, which is yeast (a type of one-celled fungus) that is used in the baking of some breads and the fermentation of certain alcohol. If you are allergic to baker's or brewer's yeast, it would cause the same symptoms as any other allergic reaction, including the possibility of anaphylaxis.

In addition to the possibility of having an allergic reaction to the baker's or brewer's yeast in alcoholic beverages, you could also be allergic to the sulfites within the alcohol. Sulfites are naturally produced within alcohol as part of the fermentation process and, like baker's or brewer's yeast, can be the catalyst for a range of allergic reactions, including anaphylaxis. In fact, sulfite allergy is so prevalent that if a product contains more than ten parts per million, then the U.S. labeling laws require manufacturers to list that the product contains sulfites.[5] Again, we will go into more detail in a later chapter about food product labels, but for now you can see how important it is to have all of your wits about you when it comes to drinking.

In no way is the preceding information meant to deter you from having a good time and drinking socially when you are of age to do so, but you do need to be fully aware of all of the risks that drinking poses, especially when it comes to your food allergies. Additionally, when you are of age to drink, you also need to consider the fact that certain alcohols, especially mixed drinks, may contain allergens directly in the drink, including some from the top eight. For instance, certain gins or vodkas can be infused with nuts or fruits. Some drinks, such as a Bloody Mary, require Worcestershire sauce, which contains fish as part of the ingredients. Other drinks, such as a piña colada, contain milk. Egg might be included in certain drinks as well. You should also be aware that certain liqueurs, such as Frangelico or amaretto, may contain nuts. Sometimes liqueurs are used as an ingredient in signature dessert coffees at restaurants, which is something that you will want to keep in mind as well.

When you are of age to drink and are ordering certain drinks at the bar, you also need to keep in mind what type of atmosphere you will be in. Most bars are loud, are filled with dim lighting, and have a lot of patrons. Bartenders are extremely busy trying to push drinks out to customers while trying to keep everyone happy. One bar may use a certain type of gin that contains nuts while another one does not. If the bar is busy, substitutions may be frequent and bartenders may have to add certain ingredients spur of the moment. Additionally, garnishes for drinks or even bowls of nuts may be in the bar. If bartenders are super busy, they are not going to wash their hands every time they are preparing a different drink, which means they could have residue on their hands containing your allergen. If you suffer from a lot of food allergies, please keep this in mind and maybe stick to simple drinks where you request the brand name of the alcohol if you know it is safe for you, stick to a bar where you know the bartender, or refrain from

It Happened to Me:
A Note from the Author Regarding Drinking

When you do reach the legal drinking age, it is completely possible to go out and enjoy yourself. As I mentioned before, I have multiple food allergies and among those allergies is baker's/brewer's yeast, which means that along with my other allergies, I am allergic to alcohol. Although I am allergic and often refrain as much as possible from eating or drinking anything while at a bar, my allergies do not stop me from going out to bars with my friends. I can have fun just like everyone else.

One experience in particular drove this point home for me. I was out for one of my best friend's bachelorette parties. My friends and I were at a small bar and, of course, chatting ensued between the bachelorette party members and a group of guys. Drinks were being bought all around, and one of the guys came over to me to ask what I was drinking because he noticed I was the only one not having anything. I explained that I didn't want to drink; I was allergic. He didn't press any further, but asked me if there was anything that I could have, including Coca-Cola or water. He actually asked in a kind manner and was not making fun of me. I replied that I could have both. The next thing I knew, he went to the bartender, who placed about ten large glasses of Coke on the bar. He told me to enjoy. When I thanked him and told him that it wasn't necessary and that there was no way that I could drink all ten, he just replied to share them with my friends and we wished each other a good night. That really meant so much to me because I realized that while drinking socially is definitely fun, just because I couldn't drink didn't mean that I couldn't enjoy myself. I learned that I belonged at a bar, a restaurant, or a party for that matter, just as much as anyone else.

"My friends ask me if I feel like I'm missing out because I can't eat anything with dairy. I tell them no because I can eat dairy-free cheese, ice cream, and cake. Pretty much anything they can eat I can eat too."—Emily C.[d]

drinking at the bar altogether. Again, it is very important to always keep yourself safe. Though it may seem like a hassle, it is very possible to hang out and to have a good time even if you are not the one drinking.

Although it is ultimately your responsibility to make sure you are safe and to be aware of your environment when it comes to your food allergies, this is where it is also vitally important to have a trusted friend with you or someone who is on board with you when it comes to your food allergies. You can discuss any concerns you have and make plans together; that way everyone can be on the same page and you can be sure to have a good time.

Your friends are there to support you and to help you along your journey, but as mentioned before, sometimes they may not be aware of everything you are feeling or of some of the concerns you may have. Make sure you talk to them about any apprehensions you may have, both now as a teenager and when you are older and go out to bar crawls together along with other parties. Maybe you will have slight anxiety about going to a new place. Maybe once you all turn the legal drinking age, you will be the official group chauffeur because you cannot drink when you go out or you cannot drink at all because of your allergies. You may wind up feeling like you are invited out just to drive everyone around. If this does happen, your friends will want to know how you are feeling, so be sure to talk it over with them. More than likely, it will not be their intention to make you feel this way and they will want to know about it.

As you get older, schedules get filled quickly and your circle of friends could change and expand, but no matter who your trusted friends are, be sure that you extend your appreciation. They are most likely always looking out for you both now and in the future, have your back in social situations, and may eat out at the same safe restaurants for you on more occasions than they would care to. Appreciation goes a long way even if you have been friends for a while. It is a great feeling to have that extra support from your friends.

Now that you have your friends and family on board with you with regard to your food allergies, it is time to start expanding your world even further. Cast your food allergy support net even wider and create a support system of those people who can help you maintain a fulfilling lifestyle, including a social calendar filled with parties.

6

CREATING YOUR CREW

....

Now that you have your family and friends on board with you in regard to your needs, as discussed in the last couple chapters, it is now time to pick up the rest of your crew and expand your world living with food allergies. Although you may come into contact with a multitude of different people over the course of any given day, not every single person who crosses your path needs to become part of your crew. However, the same people may pop up during your day-to-day activities, including teachers, coaches, neighbors, bosses at your after-school or weekend job, workers at the local market, and even your hair stylist or barber. Since you are in regular contact with these people and food allergens are most likely present during your interactions, these individuals will make great additions to your crew. It is both beneficial and necessary to tell them about your allergies and what to do if an emergency situation were to occur.

Take a moment and think about your schedule on a typical day. More than likely, you are probably realizing that during a regularly scheduled day, you see your teachers, school staff, and coaches almost as much as your family and friends. Therefore, it is extremely important to make sure that these people are on your crew. It is equally important to keep an open dialogue between school staff and coaches in relation to your needs.

School Policies

While some states and many school districts have their own policies regarding how to deal with students with food allergies, there was no uniform guideline available to school systems until 2013. As a result of the Food and Drug Administration's Food Safety Modernization Act of 2011, which focused on improving the safety of food within the United States, the Centers for Disease Control published *Voluntary Guidelines for Managing Food Allergies in Schools and Early Care and Education Programs* on October 30, 2013. Although these guidelines are not mandatory, they serve as a tool to support schools and school staff in how to administer food allergy action plans as well as improve upon plans that are already in place. The guidelines reinforce the need for food allergy education and awareness among school staff. Additionally, the guidelines stress the importance of not only having protocols in place during emergencies but also teaching people how to prevent emergency situations.[1]

While these guidelines are extremely helpful and offer some wonderful tips, the important thing to remember is in the title of the guidelines: they are voluntary. Just because they are out there, it does not mean that each school has to abide by them. They are guidelines; they are not law. With that being said, there are federal laws and regulations that support students with food allergies. Section 504 of the Rehabilitation Act of 1973 and the Americans with Disabilities Act of 1990 are two such laws, and you may already be familiar with them if you already have a plan in place at your school. In simple terms, these laws reinforce that if a school is receiving funding from the U.S. Department of Education, then it must provide equal opportunities to all students, even if some of those students have disabilities. Under these laws, a student is considered to have a disability if he or she has a physical or mental impairment that substantially limits a major life activity such as eating, breathing, or the proper functioning of bodily systems.[2]

Some people, maybe even you, find it difficult to equate food allergies with a disability. For some reason, there is a negative connotation with the word *disability*. For some people who do not fully understand the scope of food allergies or living with multiple food allergies, it may seem far-fetched to consider food allergies as a disability. After all, there is a surefire way to not suffer from an allergic reaction: avoid those foods that cause an allergic reaction. Don't eat the foods that cause a reaction, and there should never be a problem, right? *Wrong!* If only it were that simple. Of course there are different degrees of disabilities, and disabilities range in symptoms and outcomes. If you have to significantly alter your life through no choice of your own because you are limited in performing a major life activity, then you are considered to have a disability under Section 504 and the Americans with Disabilities Act. Does this mean that you cannot go about living your life? No, of course not. Does this mean that people or school staff need to treat you differently? Again, no, of course not, but they do need to take your health into consideration and accommodate you accordingly. It's the same as if you are sitting a few rows back from the board and find yourself scrunching your eyes to see. You would most likely raise your hand and let the teacher know that the board looks blurry and that you are having a difficult time seeing. Your teacher would probably move you to a seat closer to the board and then let your parent or guardian know that you may need a visit to the eye doctor. An appointment is made, glasses are purchased, and you are able to read the board just fine and resume your life as a student. Accommodations were made in order for you to be able to see the board correctly. Maybe your seat change caused another classmate to move his seat, but all the students need to be able to see the board and have the same chance to learn, so no hard feelings, right? The same holds true if you have a food allergy. Whether you like it or not, accommodations need to be made for you if you have a food allergy. Of course these accommodations need to be within reason and are put into place to keep you healthy and safe. It is ultimately up to you to ensure your own safety and well-being. For instance, if you are purchasing lunch at the cafeteria and you are unsure of the ingredients, it is up to you to ask the cafeteria staff about the food in question.

This is also a good reminder to have open communication with any member of the school staff you have regular contact with, be it the cafeteria workers, teachers, or even a school bus driver. This conversation stresses the importance of having a plan in place. If you attend a public school, these plans could fall under the 504 plan or an individualized education plan. However, if you attend a school that is not federally funded, then an emergency care plan or individualized health care plan should be implemented. Any plan would need to originate from your doctor or allergist in conjunction with you and your parents, grandparents, or guardians and be followed through with your school. As you get older, you should also take a more active role in not only understanding your plan but also knowing what should go into your plan, such as addressing different locations in school, where your auto-injectors should be kept, and so on. By taking an active interest in what is going into your plan or even putting a plan into place, you are showing that you are willing and able to take on more responsibilities. This will work out well for you because if you can show that you are taking an active role in managing your food allergies and that you can handle responsibility with regard to your allergies, more responsibilities will be given to you in general.

Adding to Your Crew

Now that you have your family, friends, and school staff on board as your crew, it is time to add a few more people and continue to cast out the safety net. No matter what the circumstances, it is always a good practice to get to know your neighbors. You do not need to become best friends, especially if there is a large age gap, but it is always nice to have additional people looking out for you and you for them. Say, for instance, you were home watching your younger sibling and for whatever reason, you found yourself having an allergic reaction with telltale signs of it turning into anaphylaxis. After calling 9-1-1 and administering your EpiPen, your younger sibling would be able to run next door and grab a neighbor for help. Your neighbor would be able to contact your parents or guardian and would take care of your younger sibling while paramedics are taking care of you. Additionally, it would be a good idea to let your neighbor know in advance where your medications are stored in case of an emergency, as well as a general idea of the foods you are allergic to. The same holds true if you are working at a job after-school or on the weekends.

If you have multiple food allergies, chances are you do not work at a restaurant or ice cream shop. More than likely, your job has nothing to do with food. However, no matter where you work, there is always a chance of an allergic reaction by foods being cross-contaminated or from something someone else brings in. In the off chance that something were to happen, you would want to inform your manager or supervisor about your allergies and where you store your auto-injectors in case of an emergency. As mentioned before, accidents can and, unfortunately, will happen. For that reason, it is best to be prepared.

Hidden Ingredients

So now that you have your family, friends, neighbors, and bosses in your crew, what about your hair stylist or barber? Why would these people have any need to know about your food allergies? Very good question; here is the answer. If you suffer from nut, soy, wheat, or milk allergies, you need to tell your hair stylist or barber because these ingredients are commonly used in shampoos, conditioners, and other hair products. Although your allergies are labeled as "food allergies," it is extremely important to remember that allergens are not solely bound to food. Certain makeup, lotions, and personal hygiene items may also contain allergens, which is why it is so important to read labels. For instance, when shopping at the local pharmacy for toothpaste and mouthwash, read the labels. Some of these products contain egg, soy, and nuts. How to read labels will be discussed in greater length in chapter 10, so for now, let's go back to your hair stylist or barber. If you are allergic to soy, for instance, be aware that there are entire lines of hair products that have soy as the main ingredient. Since you would not be ingesting the soy, it most likely would not cause an anaphylactic attack, but an allergic reaction, such as breaking out into hives, could occur. Why go through the hassle or create unnecessary anxiety around whether you may break out in hives or a rash? Additionally, why would you waste the stylist's time and your money for a wash, cut, and blow dry when you will just go home and wash your hair anyway? Know which products you are able to use, and communicate that to your hair stylist or barber. The same can hold true if you go shopping at your local supermarket and ask about ingredients at the deli, the bakery, and so on. If this is a place you frequently go to, it will be sure to accommodate you. Additionally, if your hair stylist, your barber, or the workers at the local market are taking care of you in regard to keeping you safe, you will tell other people about how wonderful they are and this will generate more business for them.

Your world is getting bigger and bigger and so is your crew, but there is an important group of people who need to be added in addition to those who come into contact with you on a daily basis. This group is probably the most important group to get on board: your doctor and medical care team.

Doctors Should Not Be People to Fear

Gone are the days when if you got sick, you contacted the local doctor who serviced the entire town and had been in practice for the last fifty years. This same doctor probably delivered your parents as well as your grandparents and it was most likely unheard of to question his diagnosis. Discussions about one's health were not the norm, and possible conditions were most likely diagnosed from a list straight out of a textbook. Why was that the case? Embarrassment about having something that was not so clear-cut? Fear of asking doctors questions? Possibly. Whatever the reason, this hands-off approach to a person's health is ending. Doctors should not be people to fear; they should be seen as confidantes and advocates for your health. Some doctors have literally seen you inside and out, so it should not be seen as weird or uncommon to talk about how you are feeling with regard to your care. Additionally, it is more important now than ever for you to build your own relationship with your medical care team.

As a teenager, you are already beginning to make certain decisions on your own, and you are becoming more self-sufficient. With that being said, many teenagers, you included, may still see a pediatrician up until college graduation. Your pediatrician was most likely chosen by a parent or guardian when you were too young to remember. When it came to your health, your parents, grandparents, or guardians were the ones to set up your appointments and speak on your behalf. As you get older, it is important to speak up for yourself. Of course, the love and support of your family is always welcome, but you should now be able to communicate with any doctor about your own health.

Well, what happens if you feel as though you cannot communicate with your doctor? Maybe your doctor was great for when you were younger, but now you feel as though she is not quite listening to your concerns. Maybe you never really got warm and fuzzy feelings from her, but your parents or guardians had a good relationship with that doctor and you never thought to question it. Now is the time to ask questions and take a more active role in your health, such as choosing another doctor.

While doctors are able to perform wonderful deeds and do amazing things in order to keep you healthy, they are still people. They have their own families, their own interests, and their own personalities. As you get older and your views and ideas change, you may recognize that you do not feel comfortable with your pediatrician or other members of your medical care team and that your personalities just do not mesh anymore. Guess what? That is OK. If this describes you, then you should begin discussing your concerns with your parents or other family first and remember to "calm-municate." As mentioned in the chapter about calm-municating, bring your concerns to your parents, grandparents, or guardians in a calm manner, making valid points about how you are feeling. Again, it is very difficult to dismiss someone's feelings if he or she is making logical points in a calm tone. Although you are more self-sufficient as a teenager, you still need to run things by your parents and/or other decision makers in your family, and if you are unhappy with the doctors providing your medical care, you can work together with your family to ensure you create a medical care team that is right for you. This also holds true if you are seeing a doctor or an allergist for the first time.

For instance, maybe you have a great relationship with your pediatrician or general practitioner who recently diagnosed you as being allergic. Your pediatrician or general practitioner then recommends you see an allergist for further testing to ensure you receive proper and appropriate medical care. Not only does your doctor recommend this allergist, but the allergist comes "highly" recommended with accolades from every major medical journal for research on allergies and immunological therapies. This allergist you are about to see is the "best in the business," and appointment wait times can be months, but you got in with only having to wait a few weeks. You feel like a VIP and in very good hands, until you actually have a face-to-face meeting with the allergist. The allergist seems to hurry you along, not really listening to all of your concerns. The best piece of advice he has for you is to stay away from everything you are allergic to and keep your auto-injector on you at all times and you should be fine. You go to make a follow-up appointment and have to wait at least a month because he is giving a talk about his research. It is wonderful that this allergist is on the cutting edge of research with regard to food allergies. Although research is extremely important and necessary in order to help all those suffering from food allergies, you may want an allergist who is more readily accessible. Having a vast knowledge base and being on the forefront of research is amazing and necessary, but keeping a practice with actual patients who experience food allergies firsthand instead of speaking to an audience of medical students is something else entirely.

You need to create an allergy action plan. This plan encompasses everything that you and others need to know in order to keep you safe and living well with regard to your food allergies. More importantly, it is a plan that you need to feel completely comfortable with, so go over it in detail as many times as you need to with your allergist or a nurse who works with your allergist. This plan will also morph into your 504 plan, emergency care plan, or individualized health plan to be implemented at your school. Some people may not care if their allergist connects with them on an emotional level or if their personalities mesh as long as the allergist knows what she is doing, but if you are one of those people who do care, it is absolutely, positively, without a doubt OK. Do not feel that you are asking too much or that you will be seen as bothersome. This is your health and your life. Your mother, father, grandmother, grandfather, brother, sister, friend, neighbor (the list can go on and on) are not the ones who have to feel comfortable with the allergist, or any other doctor for that matter; it is you. These same people are not the ones who have to carry around medication in case of an allergic reaction; it is you. These people in your life are not the ones who experience the symptoms of an allergic reaction from a food; it is you. You have a responsibility and owe it to yourself to be completely comfortable with those in charge of your medical care. Be in the know when it comes to your health and well-being. Do

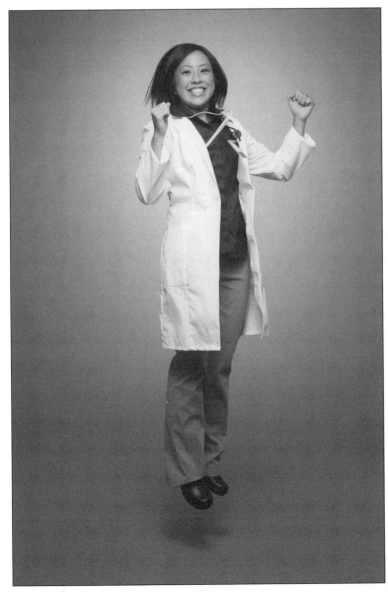

Your doctor should be one of your biggest cheerleaders. Make sure you are comfortable with your medical care team.

not find yourself saying, "Oh no!" with a list of the should haves, would haves, could haves. Do not be passive; be active! You are getting older now and should be able to start advocating for yourself without having to fall back on your parents or guardians, although their opinions should be taken into consideration. Maybe your parents have asked your allergist questions and feel comfortable with the care you are receiving or the tests that you are about to take, but you still have other concerns. This is the time to speak up, especially if the answers to your questions prompt follow-up questions. These follow-up questions, which your parents or guardians may not be able to be answer, should be asked of the allergist. Not getting an answer that may only take a minute of your allergist's time might have you waiting until your next appointment and could become a source of anxiety for you. Do not let this happen. Questions and open dialogue about your physical and emotional problems are encouraged in the medical community and should be welcome among anyone who is in your crew. There is a greater focus now on going to a doctor not only when you are sick, but also when you are healthy.

Well Visits

Seeing a doctor during a regularly scheduled healthy visit is known as a "well visit." For teenagers and adults, these well visits are much like the checkups you received as young children. During these checkups you were weighed, your height was measured, and you probably received your immunizations. At the end of the visit, you would be rewarded with lollypops and stickers. Well visits are also important as you get older so that you remain in optimal health by regularly checking in with your doctor so that in the off chance something does go wrong it can be caught early.

Additionally, if you are a person suffering from food allergies, it is always a good idea to keep your doctor abreast of how you are doing. Not only do doctors encourage this good rapport, but insurance companies are now following suit by promoting coverage for well visits and preventative care. If you think about it, promoting coverage for well visits and preventative care actually keeps costs down for the insurance companies. Being proactive about well visits will address medical issues before such issues get out of control, which would wind up being more costly for both the insurance company and you as the patient.

Primary Care and Insurance Coverage

If you are not familiar with insurance plans, there are several different types offered. Although there are plenty of plans as well as different insurance companies, a common factor in many plans, and one that is the lowest out-of-pocket expense for the patient, is that a person has one primary care physician who coordinates her care. If there is a medical issue, then the primary care physician will refer the patient to a specialist. In the case of someone suffering from food allergies, especially if there was no prior history of such an allergy, a person would bring an allergic episode such as hives to her or his primary care physician to first diagnose the cause. The doctor would ask when the hives occurred and if anything was done differently, such as a change in laundry detergent, using different soaps, or introducing different foods into the diet. Once there is evidence or a suggestion of food allergy, the patient would be given a referral to an allergist within the primary care physician's network of other medical care providers. This can be extremely helpful because your primary care physician is within the same network as your soon-to-be allergist, and both can access your medical record easily and often and keep everyone who treats you up-to-date. Additionally, if your medical care providers are all within the same facility, they generally have an on-site pharmacy and they can simply make a phone call to their pharmacy concerning potential allergens in medications that may be prescribed instead of leaving that up to you, the patient, if you were to pick it up at a local pharmacy.

Since your primary care physician is coordinating your care, it is extremely important for you to have an open and honest dialogue with him. Although you may be seeing the allergist way more than your primary care physician, you still need everyone to be to be on board with your concerns, your viewpoint, and your needs. Some people think that they may not need to have a great relationship with their primary care physician. This is false. Since this doctor will be responsible for coordinating your care, he is your first line of defense in potential health problems and your first point of contact to helping you get better. These types of plans are generally known as health maintenance organizations, or HMOs. Of course there are other types of plans, and some of them, typically known as preferred provider organizations, or PPOs, allow a person to choose any doctor or specialist she wants. If the provider is in the network, it is generally less expensive than if the provider is out of the network. Although there are many different types of plans, the overall message remains the same: there should be open communication between you, the patient, and any provider that treats you. Additionally, technology and social media have made communication between you, the patient, and your providers even easier.

Patient Portals Online

Many practices now have internal, secure websites, where patients can access their medical information. If you were to log onto these sites, you would be able

Best Allergy Sites

A great website to try is Best Allergy Sites (www.bestallergysites.com), which is a one-stop shop with a directory of allergists, companies, products, and more that would be helpful to anyone suffering from allergies or intolerances. It was created by Ruth Lovett-Smith, who began compiling a list of helpful information when her own child was diagnosed with food allergies. Best Allergy Sites is a great resource whether you have been newly diagnosed or if you have been living with allergies for a long time. Ms. Lovett-Smith wishes to spread allergy awareness and to also reiterate to those suffering from food allergies to embrace their allergies and not be embarrassed by them.[a]

to see information from prior visits, test results, and future appointments. Some of these sites also allow you to chart certain results so that you can check on your health trends. Many of these sites also allow you to send nonurgent e-mails to the provider for general health questions or to ask if an appointment may be needed. Of course it is always important to remember that if you think you may be having an allergic reaction, do not wait for a response to an e-mail. Follow the advice of your doctor and call 9-1-1. Never hesitate in an emergency or post something to a discussion forum if you need to call for an ambulance or you are unsure about using your auto-injector. However, if you do have general questions or want to expand your connections in the allergy community, you can do so at the touch of your smartphone or by going online.

If you are ever feeling down about your allergies or feel like there is no one else who understands, get yourself online. With that being said, you should always keep open communication with your parents or guardians about the sites or various forums that you would like to explore. As with anything, there are positives and negatives to going online and using social media. If you go online on your computer, smartphone, or tablet, pull up any search engine and type in "food allergies." A number of websites will pop up, and you can begin your journey into navigating the food allergy waters.

The trick is to get information from trusted sources, and a great place to start would be to ask your allergist about groups and organizations that you can join. When I spoke with Dr. David Stukus regarding the use of the Internet to gather

Some Useful Smartphone Apps

1. AllergyEatsMobile, which locates allergy-friendly restaurants and peer reviews of those restaurants. It also includes nutritional data.

2. Food Allergy Detective, which allows you to track and analyze the foods you are eating. If you find that you experience certain symptoms after eating a particular food, this app will allow you to track those symptoms. In turn, it will show trends of these symptoms in correlation to the foods that you have eaten, which you can then bring to your allergist to help diagnose your allergies.

3. Cook IT Allergy Free, which provides over two hundred allergy-friendly recipes. It also provides ingredients for safe substitutions.

4. Find Me Gluten Free, which locates gluten-free-friendly restaurants and markets.

5. Allergy and Gluten Free Scanner, which has a database of over two hundred thousand products in the United States and indicates if those products contain allergens or gluten. It also provides a list of alternative foods.

6. AroundMe allows you to locate the closest hospitals and pharmacies both nationally and internationally.

7. Content Checked, which allows you to scan the barcode of a product and see if there are any ingredients you would be allergic to based on criteria you already have programmed into the app.

information and support for food allergy sufferers, he mentioned the fact that you should

always consider the source of information, which may not be easy to determine. Most sites are not written by doctors or properly trained allergy specialists. It doesn't mean that they are unreliable, but proceed with caution as they may not relay accurate or up-to-date information. Our understanding of food allergies is changing all the time as new research gets published in medical journals. This often creates confusion, especially when interpreted incorrectly or not fully understood. Make sure that your source of information is up-to-date.

One of the best uses of the Internet for food allergies is in finding support groups. There is a wonderful network of very helpful people who devote their time and energy in helping those newly diagnosed or anyone struggling with food allergies. It can be comforting and helpful to know that there are so many others out there, and within easy reach through social media, who can help. In addition, if any site that provides information is also trying to sell you something, then, by definition, they have a conflict of interest. I would recommend extreme caution in using their information reliably. The Internet can be an excellent resource to gain a better understanding of health conditions, which can help you come up with good questions to ask your doctor. Maintaining a personal relationship with your doctor, who understands what makes you unique, is always the most important part of establishing a correct diagnosis and treatment.[3]

Helpful Organizations

There are a number of great organizations that you should consider becoming a member of. For instance, one such organization is Food Allergy Research & Education (FARE), which is a 501(c)(3) nonprofit organization that was created in 2012 by two previous groups (Food Allergy and Anaphylaxis Network and Food Allergy Initiative). It focuses on providing evidence-based education and resources as well as promoting awareness and advocacy.[4] Another great organization that was formed in 2014 is the Food Allergy & Anaphylaxis Connection Team (FAACT). FAACT is a wonderful resource for education, awareness, outreach, and emotional support for those affected by food allergies.[5]

Both FAACT and FARE have specific sections on their websites devoted to teenagers living with food allergies and offer advice to teens from teens through special advisory groups and Facebook support groups. Be sure to check these out and maybe even offer some advice for others based on your personal experiences. Both of these organizations also sponsor special teen conferences during the year where, if you attend, you will meet with other teens to discuss how to live well with food allergies. The conferences provide breakout sessions for you to meet in small groups to discuss certain topics when dealing with food allergies. They also offer breakout sessions for siblings and parents of those with food allergies. If you are able to attend one of these conferences, it would not only be a great learning experience for you, but you would be able to meet other teens just like you and create valuable friendships that could last a lifetime. To get more information about possible teen conferences, be sure to check out both FAACT's and FARE's websites.

In addition to FAACT and FARE, another useful organization is the Asthma and Allergy Foundation of America, which offers resources for patients, caregivers, and health care professionals. The Asthma and Allergy Foundation of America has local chapters that you can join based upon the region of the country that you live in. Each chapter has its own events and support groups, and if you decide to become a member, you will be expanding your network of people within the food allergy community. Remember that you are never alone.

In addition to the actual websites of these organizations and joining their Facebook pages, you can also follow these organizations on Pinterest or Twitter. Twitter is very useful in this regard because it offers you suggestions based on the people you already follow. You may also find yourself reading the tweets or retweets of the people you follow. In doing so, you will probably find that you have come across another member connected to the food allergy community and begin following her as well; it is more than likely that all of these people are trusted sources or sources of support within the food allergy community. Additionally, you will find doctors and allergists on Twitter, including Dr. David Stukus. He tweets often and had this to say about Twitter:

I have always been a supporter of patient education and public awareness but started becoming more and more frustrated with all of the misinformation available on the Internet. I wanted to provide a source of reliable information that people could turn towards to help answer questions.

As I've "found my voice," I've learned that I can have a lot of fun with Twitter. It is a wonderful way to interact with the rest of the world. In addition to providing evidence based information, I can let my followers see my personality a bit as well. After all, I am a pediatrician at heart and love working with families and children. I also interact with allergists and doctors from all over the world, which educates me—I've learned a ton.

I am a strong believer that more providers should use social media to engage with the public, as well as their own patients. I have become a better doctor just by being an active Twitter user. I am more aware of the issues and concerns shared by parents and patients, which helps me ask appropriate questions or provide more support in the office. I have also been able to network and meet new people, which has opened up new avenues for me to increase public awareness. And lastly, being limited to 140 characters has really changed the way I provide information. It's really challenging to put medical information into a 140-character tweet, but that forces me to stay focused and trim any excess information that really isn't necessary to begin with.

I encourage all teenagers with food allergies to use the Internet and social media to explore and find others with similar food allergies or personalities. Everyone is different in how they cope with their food allergies and manage avoidance on a daily basis. It's definitely not "one size fits all" and that's where the variety found on the Internet can be so helpful.

The really nice part is that you can still interact and learn while remaining anonymous. You can share as little or as much information about yourself as you are comfortable with. Explore the many faces of food allergy and hear their personal stories. Eventually, you will connect with someone that you feel comfortable with. Many people have used social media to find others in their community, which can lead to actual face to face groups or events and a whole new support network.[6]

Food Allergy Coaches

In addition to finding allergists or other doctors who use social media, you may find an entire group of people who would be great additions to either connect with occasionally or to join your crew. These people are food allergy coaches. What is a food allergy coach, you may ask? Well, think of a sports coach who specializes in helping those in the food allergy community. More often than not, a food allergy coach is someone with a firsthand experience of dealing with food allergies and the effects they can have on someone's life. To find out more about what a food allergy coach does, let's talk to two coaches.

The first coach, Kristin Beltaos, MA, owner of a Gift of Miles, where she provides coaching/consulting services, had this to say about coaching:

Psychologists and psychiatrists focus on the diagnosis and the treatment of mental disorders, such as anxiety, depression, dysfunctions, obsessions, compulsiveness, or a feeling that they are not functioning to capacity, etc. Moreover, therapy is about healing wounds of the past. Although I will say that many in this field have evolved their clinical practices to include coaching; it's actually a very natural progression.

With regard to coaching/consulting, for many healthy individuals coaching/consulting begins when a new skill set needs to be acquired, like trying to find your footing and a "new normal" after the diagnosis of life-threatening food allergies or needing an advocate to assist in the establishment of your Individual Healthcare Plan and/or 504 Plan at school. For others it's when we are stuck in a rut: in a job, in a relationship, or trying to gain balance amidst life's daily grind or chaos. Sometimes we need help to propel ourselves and grow beyond, gain balance, and restructure our lives.

I am of the thought that everyone should have a coach. Even coaches should have coaches/consultants! I say this because it's a relationship that can be resurrected whenever you need it. There are so many positives to utilizing a coach; here are a few:

1. Because of technology, coaching/consulting can be done from anywhere: in-person and via telephone, video conferencing, and even e-mail.
2. The collaborative and synergistic relationship between a coach/consultant and client sets a client up for success with well-defined goals, deadlines that support growth, accountability necessary to complete assignments, and progress toward goals and attainment of your objectives.
3. But most importantly, coaching provides a client with the emotional support that is lacking in his/her life, especially when friends, family, and society don't always understand.

When it comes to food allergy awareness, Kristin provides the following programs in her home state of Minnesota as she is a licensed trainer with the Minnesota Center for Professional Development. Part of her training is to teach food allergy continuing education to early childhood and school-age providers and educators:

I provide onsite-sponsored trainings and in-person trainings through Think Small(www.thinksmall.org). My courses are also offered online through Eager-to-Learn (www.eagertolearn.org) and a part of the professional development resources with the Minnesota Association for the Education of Young Children and the Minnesota School-Age Care Alliance (Minnesota AEYC-SACA). The in-person courses are

• Caring for Food Allergic Children in an Early Childhood Care Environment. This training provides guidance on how to handle daily care, manage safety, and promote inclusiveness of food allergic children. You'll learn about food allergies and intolerances, the identification, treatment, and medication management of allergic reactions. Create a parent/care provider partnership based on mutual responsibility and respect that ensures the safety of all allergic children.
• Food Allergic Plans of Protection: Demystifying Food Allergy Policy/Guidelines, 504 and Individual Health Plans. This training provides guidance to school/district personnel on how to formulate comprehensive food allergy (fa) policy/guidelines, develop individualized, fa

Health Plans and/or 504 plans, and build an Awareness Communication Program to keep fa on the top of the minds of all stakeholders. Understand the dangers, the prevention, identification, and treatment of an allergic reaction.

- Diminish Food Allergy Bullying with Inclusiveness. This training provides strategies on how to create an inclusive environment by minimizing the spotlight of difference, teach appreciation, compassion, and tolerance to children and formulate a zero tolerance policy with consequences, based on age, for food allergy bullying.

The online courses are available nationally and internationally:

- Food Allergy Facts, Fibs & Fundamentals. This training provides guidance on food allergies, understanding the facts and dispelling the myths. You'll learn the difference between a food allergy and an intolerance, how to read ingredient and manufacturing labels, what is cross contamination, the sneaky places where allergens can hide and have a better understanding of parents of food allergic children. This course also offers a question and answer session with the instructor so that you may get your individual food allergy questions answered.
- Treatment & Management of Food Allergy Anaphylaxis. This training provides guidance on how to assess and treat allergic reactions of food allergic children. You'll learn about the identification, treatment, and medication management of allergic reactions and anaphylaxis.
- Food Allergy Management: It's a Partnership. This training provides guidance on how to develop the necessary guidelines, policies, and procedures to ensure safety and inclusion on a daily basis. This course also discusses food allergy bullying and how to teach compassion. Taking this and the prerequisite courses will result in educated providers who are able to offer enormous comfort and security to parents of food allergic children.

Lastly, I also speak at a variety of conferences throughout the year, to name a few: Education Minnesota, Minnesota Early Childhood Educator's Conference, Minnesota AEYC-SACA Annual Conference, and the Provider's Choice Conference.

With regard to living well with food allergies, Kristin suggests, "Create the kind of community that we want to live in and surround yourself with people that inform, support, and most of all like to have fun and find the humor in our sometimes challenging lives, but most importantly, we are all more than the challenges that we manage."[7] To find out more about Kristin and her programs you can go to her website, www.agiftofmiles.com.

Now it is time to hear from another food allergy coach, Sloane Miller. In addition to being an accomplished writer with an award-winning blog, *Please Don't Pass the Nuts,* and a critically acclaimed book, *Allergic Girl: Adventures in Living Well with Food Allergies,* Sloane is also the owner of Allergic Girl Resources, Inc., providing food allergy coaching services. When asked to go into a little more detail as to her role as a food allergy coach, Sloane had this to say:

> As someone who has had food allergies, asthma, allergies, and eczema her entire life, and a licensed psychotherapeutic social worker, I'm uniquely qualified to offer support, guidance, advice, and referrals for our community.
>
> My role as a food allergy counselor and coach is to support kids, teens, parents, adults who are managing food allergies; to help them build upon the strengths they already have and work towards the goals that they devise, whether it's traveling to a distant location or leaning how to be a better advocate for their medical needs with schools, friends, or family.
>
> In short, as a food allergy counselor and coach I support clients as they create their own transformations towards their best lives while managing severe life threatening food allergies.[8]

If you have not picked up a copy of Sloane's book, you should do so as it is another great resource in learning to live well with food allergies. In addition to her writing accomplishments, Sloane has also been instrumental in liaising between figures in the restaurant industry and the food allergic community. Sloane comments that although she has food allergies, she is

> a huge foodie; I love food and dining out. It was only natural that as menus and restaurant trends change (more tree nuts, more fish, more hidden ingredients on menus) I needed to step up my personal advocacy efforts. And what I did for myself I did for others: creating strategies, language and tools to dine out safely, effectively, and joyously.[9]

Sloane is truly one of those people who practices what she preaches, so to speak, and as a result of that, she touches on many emotions that go through someone's head in dealing with food allergies in everyday life, including anxiety about anaphylactic attacks. When discussing anxiety in relation to dealing with food allergies, Sloane advises that

> it's completely normal to feel some anxiety around food allergy reactions and/or anaphylaxis, a swift and severe allergic reaction.

Here's one way to begin to learn to separate what is an irrational fear (not a real risk with a probable outcome) versus a true concern (a true risk but manageable).

1. Write down all of your fears, anxieties, concerns, and even your worst case scenarios. Get them out of your head and onto a piece of paper or computer document.
2. Then take a long look at that list. Are there fears on there you know not to be true, actual, or possible? Are there scenarios you've heard of that make you nervous but never saw any evidence of happening? Are there medical questions that you don't know the answer to but know you should? In short, do your best to take a critical look at your concerns and begin to sort out the rational fears from the irrational ones.
3. Go over the whole list with a trusted food allergy aware friend or family member. Explore your feelings: how does it feel to write the list? What is different once you wrote down your fears? Did you gain any clarity, if so where? What is still unclear to you? How did you feel looking at your fears critically? What still is a big unknown or upsetting you?
4. If any of your fears are medical in nature, and I suspect many of them will be, make an appointment to have a consultation with your board certified medical health provider. This appointment will be all about you; you will lead it, you will ask the questions and get

Celebrities with Food Allergies

You are not in this alone. Some famous names who also suffer from food allergies are Halle Berry (actress with a shellfish allergy), Zooey Deschanel (actress with a dairy, egg, and wheat allergy), Jo Frost (Supernanny personality with a peanut, tree nut, crustacean, and rye allergy), Ben Lovett (musician and member of Mumford & Sons with a peanut allergy), Tom Poti, (NHL player with multiple food allergies), Ray Romano (actor with a peanut allergy), Billy Bob Thornton (actor with a shellfish allergy and wheat and dairy intolerance), and Serena Williams (tennis star with a peanut allergy).[b]

the answers. Never talked with your doctor before? That's okay, this is a great time to start. Write down their answers or record the conversation.

5. After your appointment, talk about what you learned with your trusted friends and family so they can support you as you process this new information.

6. Continue to extract for yourself irrational fears from rational and possible risks. Go back to your allergist's words and recommendations. Ground yourself in the reality of the risk versus your fears around the risk.

This is a broad outline of a longer exercise. In a coaching relationship with me, we would go into a deeper version of this exercise but this is a good place to start.

Please note: if you are having feelings of anxiety, depression, and they are impeding normal life functioning and enjoyment, please see a local mental health provider immediately for an evaluation.[10]

It Happened to Me:
A Note Regarding Anxiety and Food Allergies

Coming to terms with having multiple life-threatening food allergies and the lifestyle changes that come with them was very difficult for me. After I was first diagnosed, I began developing a fear of eating foods that were not prepared by either myself or my mother, and after I had my first anaphylactic attack, my anxieties increased. These anxieties increased to the point where I was afraid to eat anything while I was alone, even if it was something I knew was a safe food. Realizing that my anxieties were getting out of control, I discussed my concerns with my parents and I sought counseling. It only took a few visits for me to get control over my fears and to become actively involved in my own health and well-being. Maybe it was talking about my fears out in the open or to a person I knew would not judge me for my feelings, but it was the best thing I could have done. I made the conscious decision to not let my allergies control me, and I have not looked back since. If you suffer from anxiety because of your allergies, do not be ashamed to talk about it or seek additional support if you need it. There is nothing to be embarrassed about!

When discussing teenagers in particular, Sloane stated that the "teenage years are also a massive growing time and testing time for all teens and teens with any medical condition are not excused. Teens must test boundaries, individuate from family, create a sense of self, spread their wings." She went on to say that the important thing teenagers and parents need to remember is that "trust is created over time. You would never put a teen who has never driven a car, not even down the driveway, into a Maserati and tell her to drive on the Autobahn. Food allergy management is much the same, start with small tasks that will lead to larger independent acts."[11] To find out more about Sloane and her coaching services, please visit her website at allergicgirl.com/sloane-miller/.

In continually brushing up on your skills to advocate for yourself and expanding your world of support, you are already well on your way to creating larger, independent acts. Just like learning how to ride a bike, you started out small by speaking to your family, then you went on to spread the word to your friends. Once you had your family and friends on board, then you realized that you could reach out to create a larger support system. With this larger support system and through more connections within the food allergy community, you are casting out a wider support net and opening up your world. As your world opens up and you learn to trust more, if you have been suffering from anxiety with regard to your food allergies, you may find that your anxieties will lessen at this point. As you continue to widen your world, you may be ready to put yourself out there and learn to trust even more when you open up your world to the world of dating.

LOVE IN THE TIME OF FOOD ALLERGIES

Now that you are familiar with how to deal with your friends and going out to parties when it comes to your food allergies, there is another huge factor that you are probably worried about. Fear not. Whether you suffer from food allergies or not, the whole notion of dating can be worrisome for all teenagers. In fact, dating can be worrisome for anyone at any age, and for some people the thought of dating alone can cause hives. You would not see all of those commercials for dating websites and services, magazines offering dating advice, and numerous television shows dedicated to finding "the one" if dating came easy to everyone or if it was not something that people thought about on a frequent basis. Although

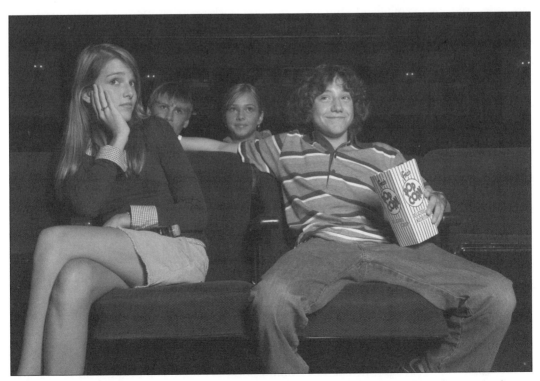

Dating can be worrisome for anyone, but it doesn't need to be awkward just because of your food allergies.

Dating Website for People with Food Allergies

There is a dating website called Singles with Food Allergies (www
.singleswithfoodallergies.com/aboutus.php) founded on the idea that
people can connect with other food allergy sufferers and not have to worry
about explaining about food allergies while on a date.

dating can be a cause for worry, it can also be a time of excitement, self-discovery, and friendships that will last a lifetime.

If you have started dating, do you remember back to your first date? It was most likely someone with whom you have gone to school or someone with whom you have grown up. If this is the case, your date most likely already knows that you have food allergies. However, it is very important to remember that just because someone is aware that your food allergies exist, it does not mean that he knows what having food allergies entails or what to do if an allergic reaction occurs. When you discuss where and what you will be doing for your date, remind the person about your food allergies. If your date is not someone you have grown up with and has no idea about your food allergy history, tell him or her about your food allergies and everything that your allergies entail. Be sure to discuss the foods that would cause an allergic reaction and that it is important for you to stay away from these offending foods. It is also important to discuss where you keep your auto-injector and demonstrate how to use it in case an emergency were to occur. After having this important discussion with your date, you may decide to go out to eat at a local restaurant you know is safe for you and where you feel comfortable with the waitstaff and the menu. However, a date should not be synonymous with dinner at a restaurant. Get creative and do something different!

There are many activities you can do that are not centered on food that would make for a great date. For instance, you could attend a show in the city, go to a local museum, take a walk in the park, take a dance class, take an art class, or go bowling. Depending on the season, there are additional activities you can take part in like ice skating in the winter or going to the beach in the summer. You could also look up fun events going on in your area during the course of the year, and you may even find a non-food-centered activity right in your hometown. The possibilities are endless! The important thing to remember is that even if you do not make a strong love connection, this person cares enough about you to want to get to know you better by going on a date. Since this person cares about you, she

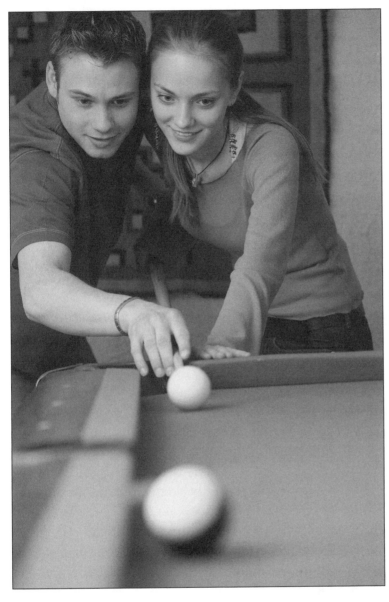

Make date night about activities and experience. Do not have it centered on food.

or he will want to make sure that you feel both safe and comfortable when you go out, so do not be shy when talking about your food allergies. Once you feel comfortable and safe, you can be free to be yourself and start focusing on having fun, which is what dating is all about. While allergies should not define who you are, they are a part of you and it is important to have this discussion with a potential date as soon as possible, especially if the potential date is going to turn into a potential kissing partner.

For example, maybe the person you went on that first date with is someone who shares a lot of your interests, and the two of you really seem to click. You have gone on one or two official dates and have been hanging out a lot in between. Not only is this person fun to be around, but he is not so bad to look at, either. You notice that each time you are together, you want to be physically closer to this person, either by holding hands or putting your arms around each other. Eventually, these actions coupled with your attraction to this person's great character will lead to your first kiss. A first kiss has the potential to be awkward, but if your potential kissing partner is not made aware of the seriousness of your food allergies or the potential for you to have a reaction, the possibility of the kiss being awkward should be the least of your worries. If your kissing partner has eaten a food you can have an allergic reaction to, it can threaten your health and safety. As mentioned earlier, a discussion about your food allergies and what that means in terms of kissing needs to be discussed as soon as possible. Additionally, depending on how sensitive you are to a reaction, your date or kissing partner will need to be aware that you may get a reaction if he touched one of your offending foods and still has residue somewhere on his skin or clothes. Certain makeups and lotions can contain milk, nuts, egg, or soy. It is also important to remember that crumbs or residue can possibly linger on facial hair, and if you are that sensitive, this can also cause an allergic reaction. It may seem like a lot to think about and a lot of information to relay to someone all at once, but it needs to be done.

Having the Food Allergy Talk

It will never seem like a good time to have "the talk," as it is often referred to in the food allergy community, so the sooner you do it, the better. It will give you relief once you have shared this information and put yourself in the position of your date. If it was your date who had the severe food allergies, you would want to know about them, right? You would want to make sure that you did everything you could to prevent your date from having an allergic reaction. Your date will almost assuredly feel the same way. So why hold this vital information in? Whether you have known your date for a long time or a short time, it is very important to discuss your food allergies. In terms of discussing them with someone you have only known for a short time, read over the following scenario.

Say, for instance, you are at a party and you see your crush from the other side of the room. Your eyes meet for a moment. You look away, but find yourself smiling and look back to find that your crush is approaching you. You begin to talk and the two of you are really starting to hit it off. You have so much in common, including some mutual friends, and your crush seems to be laughing at most of your jokes, which is always a plus. There is a slight pause in between laughs and you suddenly see your crush close his eyes and start to lean in. He is probably thinking just one thing: that right there in that moment he wants to give you a kiss. You are most likely a little anxious, a little excited, and then your nerves might start setting in. You might be thinking about everything that your crush had just eaten or could have eaten over the course of the day and start freaking out about how to handle the situation. In all honesty, this type of situation could occur frequently, and depending on how it is handled, it could definitely make for an awkward situation. However, it would be more awkward for you to kiss your crush and then suffer from an anaphylactic attack because he had a food you were severely allergic to right before or during the party.

Kissing

When you suffer from severe food allergies that can result in an anaphylactic attack, wondering what the person you are about to kiss has eaten over the course of the day does need to be a thought that crosses your mind. In fact, there actually was a kissing study done that measured the amount of time peanut protein stays in the mouth, and the results confirm that this should not be just another passing thought. This study was published in the *Journal of Allergy and Clinical Immunology* back in 2006. People who participated in the study had to eat approximately two tablespoons of peanut butter. The researchers of the study then collected the saliva of the study participants at various times to establish when the protein in the saliva diminished. Additionally, the researchers tested the saliva after the study participants cleaned their mouths using different techniques such as gum chewing and tooth brushing.[1] Dr. Jennifer Maloney, who was one of the coauthors of the 2006 study, advises that the safest approach is to have the person whom you are kissing avoid the allergen altogether. If this does not seem feasible, then based on her study, Dr. Maloney suggests the next best course of action is to wait approximately four and a half to five hours after possible ingestion of an allergen and have the nonallergic kissing partner brush her teeth vigorously beforehand.[2] Now you are probably thinking, so much for romance or a spur-of-the-moment kiss, and how could this situation not result in awkwardness? Again, remember that although you may not be able to control the situation you are faced with, you always hold the power to control your reaction to a situation.

With that being said, let us go back to the earlier scenario where your crush is leaning in for the kiss. You have no idea what this person has eaten and you really want to be able to kiss him back, so what do you do?

As with most things, there are a few ways you can approach this situation, and it completely depends on your personality and how long you have known your potential kissing partner. Chances are, if you have known each other for a while and have gone to school together, he is already aware of your food allergies and may just need a gentle reminder. If you have not gone to school with this person or he has no idea about your food allergies, then it will be a little more work on your part, but completely doable. If this is the case, you may want to handle this situation with a little humor to make it feel less awkward for both of you and to lighten the mood. Maybe your kissing partner will find what you have to say amusing, maybe not, but it could serve as an icebreaker and get the real conversation about your allergies rolling. If improvisational humor is not your thing, feel free to deliver the food allergy talk your own way or just get straight to the point. How you deliver the information is not what is important. The important thing is that you do deliver the information and stress the seriousness of a food allergic reaction if it were to occur, as well as how to help you in such a situation.

How Much Information Should You Give?

Now that you have worked up the courage and found a time where you want to discuss your food allergies, you are probably wondering exactly what you need to tell your date or potential kissing partner. You are also probably wondering how much information will be too much information, especially if this is before your very first date and the topic of restaurants comes up. You do not want to scare off your date before you even go out for the first time, and you may be having an internal conflict about giving the correct amount of information. Again, this conversation will be easier if your potential date or kissing partner is already aware of your food allergies. However, as mentioned previously, even if your date or potential kissing partner knows you have allergies, never assume that she will be aware of the initial symptoms of an allergic reaction or how to assist you in an emergency. This person would need a refresher on what you are allergic to, where you keep your auto-injectors, and how to use them if a severe reaction were to occur. If your date or potential kissing partner is unfamiliar with food allergies, then you need to have a complete conversation, not just a refresher, about what you are allergic to, where you store your auto-injectors, and how to use the auto-injectors. Additionally, depending on your comfort level with your potential date, you could go into a greater in-depth conversation about cross-contamination and the fact that food ingredients can appear in such things as makeup, lotions, and shampoos. Always answer any questions your date may have, and once you both feel more comfortable you can talk about your allergies to a greater extent. You can always gauge by the questions a nonallergic person asks if she really understands the information you are delivering, and you can also judge if she truly cares about what you are saying.

    In general, someone who asks you out on a date or someone who has a romantic interest in you will want to keep you safe and will want to know more about you. If your date does not seem to be grasping what you are saying with regard to your food allergies or seems to be making light of this information, try to keep the conversation going. It can be a lot to take in all at once, especially if this person has never had to deal with food allergies or something life threatening before. However, if this person continues to seem cavalier or even makes jokes when you are discussing something so important, then this is clearly not the right love connection for you. Although you are a teenager and in no way thinking about a lifetime partner at this point in your life, you do want to make sure that the person you date or are romantically involved with is someone who is going to take your allergies seriously and react appropriately in an emergency situation.

For a few people, the idea of your food allergies and everything that comes with them may honestly be too much for them to handle and to think about. Your personalities may mesh perfectly and you may have a lot in common, but he may not be willing to make accommodations for you when it comes to your food allergies because it seems like too much work. Instead of being upset with this person, in a way you should be thankful for his honesty. You do not want to be with someone who is not going to make accommodations for you. This is also something to consider as you get older. Once you have an established career and lifestyle as a young adult going into adulthood and are out in the dating world, the profession of your potential date may not be conducive to your food allergies. If he is in the food industry or is constantly having to attend company-sponsored dinners or outings, you may be the one who does not want to deal with having to be so constantly vigilant about preventing a reaction, and that is OK, too. Although your food allergies are just a small part of your makeup, being aware, managing your allergies, and keeping you safe are nonnegotiable when it comes to being with someone.

With that being said, you also have to make sure that you are always honest with yourself and what your comfort level is when it comes to dating with your food allergies. The important thing to always remember is that if someone cares enough about you, she will be willing to navigate your allergies with you and take the necessary precautions to keep you safe. If you are in a long-term relationship this gets easier every day.

Food Allergies and Long-Term Relationships

Once you have found someone who shares your interests and takes your allergies seriously, you may decide to start hanging out with that person more and more. Eventually this person may become your boyfriend or girlfriend, and you will find yourself in a long-term relationship. Once in such a relationship, then you will not have to discuss your allergies all the time. It will become second nature for both of you regarding what to do, what to eat, and how to use an auto-injector if an emergency were to arise. Together, you can decide on what to do for a date and to take part in activities that are not food related. Or, if you so choose, make it about food, but safe food, of course! You could decide to try cooking some allergy-friendly food together that you both can enjoy. Sometimes cooking a safe meal together is a good reinforcement on teaching your boyfriend or girlfriend how to read labels and the importance of the "May contain" statement, if there is one, on the ingredients list. It would also be beneficial to show her the importance of using different cooking utensils in order to prevent cross-contamination. Remember, as mentioned earlier, it is just like riding your bike as a child. The more practice you get sharing the practical steps of staying safe and the more frequently you take the steps to keep you safe, the easier cooking will be. The first time is always the hardest. You may find that after a while, your boyfriend or girlfriend may become more diligent than you when it comes to managing your food allergies.

For a lot of couples where one person suffers from food allergies and the other does not, the non-food-allergic partner completely avoids the foods that cause the allergic partner to suffer a reaction. If a nonallergic partner does continue to eat an offending food, he will know to eat the food well in advance of seeing the allergic partner and be sure to wash up and brush his teeth appropriately. Again, it will become second nature for both of you.

Having food allergies and being able to discuss your needs with a romantic partner also makes for a very honest relationship because you have to communicate well. Your safety and well-being depend on it. For instance, just because your girlfriend may have a latte and dulce de leche ice cream sundae knowing that you suffer from a milk allergy and then she does not want to kiss you for fear of giving you a reaction, it does not mean that she does not love you or care about you. You have to be sure to understand that your girlfriend has made accommodations for you when it comes to your food allergies, in some cases avoiding the food that can cause you to have a reaction. You also need to make accommodations for her. As you know firsthand, it can be very difficult not to eat certain foods, and she may at times want to eat food that you cannot have. As long as your safety is put first and you are made aware of what your girlfriend has eaten, then this should not be a cause of concern about your relationship. Remember that talking about your feelings, especially when it comes to discussing your allergies, is very important to any relationship. If something is bothering you, be sure to calm-municate and talk honestly about how you are feeling. Your boyfriend or girlfriend cares about you and would not want you to be upset. If you are open and honest with him or her and most importantly, with yourself, you can never go wrong. So get out there and have fun!

Let's review the dos and don'ts of dating when it comes to having food allergies:

- *Do* talk about your food allergies to your potential date or kissing partner right away.
- *Don't* wait to discuss your food allergies and don't be embarrassed about your food allergies. Although your food allergies are a small part of you, they are still a part of you.
- *Do* get creative and discuss non-food-related activities to try with your date. The focus of a date should be on having fun and getting to know someone better, not on going out to eat.
- *Don't* be afraid to answer any questions your date may have.
- *Do* show your date how to use your auto-injector in case an emergency situation occurs.
- *Don't* assume that just because your date is already aware of your food allergies that he or she knows exactly what having food allergies entails.

It Happened to Me:
A Note from the Author Regarding Relationships

As mentioned before, I was diagnosed with food allergies at the age of twenty-one, and I was lucky enough that my boyfriend was willing to stick by me. We are now married, and he has been instrumental in helping make sense of living a life together with food allergies. I think an important part of our relationship is open communication. He understands the seriousness of food allergic reactions. He tries not to eat anything I am allergic to after lunchtime so that when he comes home at the end of the day, he will not put me at risk for an allergic reaction. However, there are times when he does have things that would cause an allergic reaction for me and we cannot kiss, but in no way does this mean he loves me any less. I understand that he makes accommodations for me, and I need to make accommodations for him. For example, if my husband was looking forward to having a meal at a particular restaurant, but it is a place where I don't feel comfortable eating, I will still go and sit through the meal even if I just order a water. Additionally, my husband knows that I have my certain utensils and cleaning products that I keep separate from the rest of our family, and he tries his best to reduce cross-contamination in our kitchen. In no way do we have a perfect system and sometimes mistakes do happen, but I know that he ultimately has my best interest at heart, which is all anyone can ask for.

- *Do* be honest with yourself about your own comfort level. If something is making you uncomfortable, discuss it.
- *Don't* be afraid to be yourself! Although you do have allergies, your allergies do not define who you are. Allow your date to get to know the *you* beyond your allergies.
- *Do* go out there and have fun, including dining out at your favorite food-allergy-friendly restaurant if you so choose.

8

DINING IN OR OUT?

....

Finding Your Comfort Level

If you are a person who suffers from food allergies, when it comes to dining out, you more than likely come from one of two mind-sets, the first being that dining out is too much of a hassle and way too stressful to even bother with, especially if you suffer from multiple life-threatening food allergies, and the second being that you have no problems dining out and may in fact consider yourself a "foodie." Whichever side you may fall on or whether you find yourself somewhere in the middle, the important thing to remember is that it really depends on your own comfort level. With that being said, whether you are all for going out to eat or you are a little hesitant, know that it is completely possible to dine out with multiple food allergies, as long as you take the necessary precautions and steps to ensure your safety while eating out. This should not be a problem for you since more than likely it has become routine in everything that you do anyway. The same rules apply when you are going out to eat at a restaurant as they do when you are going to a party, except that you may need to do a little more research before you dine out, whereas you can simply attend a party.

Eating Out at a Restaurant

First and foremost, if you are thinking about going out to eat at a restaurant, remember to use your common sense. It is becoming more and more accepted that restaurants need to cater to patrons with food allergies, and many restaurants are making reasonable efforts in doing so. Depending on your allergies, the type of cuisine that is served in a particular restaurant should determine whether you go there. For instance, if you are someone who has been known to have an anaphylactic attack to fish or shellfish, it would not be wise to eat at a restaurant that predominantly serves seafood. Additionally, if you are allergic to nuts, tree nuts, or soy, it may not be in your best interest to eat at a restaurant that mainly serves Asian dishes, as a lot of these dishes contain nuts or have a soy base. If you are allergic to milk, then it would not be a good idea to go to the local ice cream shop

"I frequently go out to eat at restaurants. Most of the restaurants are very familiar with food allergies and are accommodating and will check ingredients for me. There has been only one time in the last few years where a restaurant was hesitant to serve me anything because they couldn't guarantee anything was safe for me because of cross-contamination."—Zoe P.[a]

and take your chances ordering a slush or one of the other nondairy items that might be on the list, because the risk of cross-contamination is too high. Additionally, many restaurants serve a multitude of different dishes and the variety of dishes served may contain all of the top allergens, including allergens that are not as common. If that is the case, you are probably wondering what you should do and if it really is worth the trouble of eating out. As with anything, it will take a little extra work on your part, but it can be absolutely worth the work.

As mentioned before, eating with a group of people is much more than just sharing a meal together; it is a social experience that should not be missed just because you have food allergies. When you have eliminated the obvious restaurants because those particular facilities serve your main allergen in many of their entrees, the second step is to go online. Not only do most restaurants have a website, but many restaurants also have their menus listed on their website. By looking over the menu ahead of time, you can see if there are any viable options for you and if it would be possible to change or withhold some ingredients in the dish to accommodate your food allergies.

If all looks promising, contact the restaurant and speak with a manager or chef to see if these accommodations can in fact be made for you. More than likely the restaurant will be able to cater to your food allergy needs. Even if this is agreed upon and you set a reservation time with the manager or chef, do not

The AllergyEats App

A great tool to use before eating out is the AllergyEats app where those with food allergies write about their experiences dining out and give restaurants a score. AllergyEats has now partnered with OpenTable and makes eating out with food allergies that much easier.

assume that once you arrive at the restaurant every staff member will know about your allergies and the conversation you had with the manager or chef. Kindly remind the host or hostess that you made a reservation with the manager/chef you spoke with about your food allergies, but wanted to ensure that it is still okay to eat at that restaurant. The host or hostess will relay this information to your server, and your server will confirm with the manager or chef, who, more than likely, will come out to speak to you as well. Again, when you actually place the order with your server, remind him or her about the foods you are allergic to even if you have just confirmed your allergies with the manager or chef. Although this sounds like a long and drawn-out process, in all actuality, this process will only take a few minutes, but these few minutes are very important so that you can have a safe and enjoyable dining experience.

Additionally, in order to have a safe dining experience, you should always be prepared in case of an allergic reaction. This means that you will need to bring all of your medication with you, including two auto-injectors, and wear your medical identification jewelry. You may also want to bring chef cards with you in case the server or chef wants to have a quick and easy reminder of your exact allergies. Chef cards are wallet-sized cards that you can carry, and state the fact that you have a severe food allergy, the foods you are allergic to, and what to do in an emergency. You can choose to create your own cards, or there are many card templates that are free to download on many of the food allergy advocacy sites such as Food Allergy Research & Education (FARE). Chef cards can also be downloaded in a variety of different languages and might be useful if traveling internationally. If you are not traveling internationally and are going out to eat at a restaurant in your area, you do not necessarily have to use the chef cards and hopefully will not have to use any medications, but remember that it is always better to be prepared. It may be easier for the waiter or waitress to simply hand the chef your chef card along with your requests for a special meal or to create a meal without certain ingredients. That way, the chef will have the list of what you are allergic to right in front of her or his face and readily available so the room for error is even less.

Another good rule of thumb is that if you have not eaten at a particular restaurant before or if you suffer from multiple food allergies, try to go to the restaurant during nonpeak hours. That way the risk of cross-contamination from other dishes is greatly reduced, and the staff can take more time to focus on getting your meal perfect rather than rushing to get dishes out to the many diners in a timely fashion. This is also a wonderful way to get to know the restaurant staff. If the restaurant does a great job at preparing your food and you have a positive experience, then you will more than likely be a repeat customer. Even if the staff does get to know you, be sure that no matter what, you always remind anyone who will be in contact with your food about your food allergies; it never hurts to have people be alerted and vigilant to your needs.

One Person Can Make a Difference

The legislation that passed in Rhode Island in July 2013 was the result of a teenager just like you. Danielle M. was a junior in high school with a history of food allergy to nuts as well as food allergies in her family. She reached out to Senator Louis P. DiPalma to make a change within the state of Rhode Island to allow those with food allergies the ability to dine out safely. Follow Danielle's example and realize that you can make a difference![b]

Keeping you, the customer, happy and safe is not only in your best interest, but it is also in the best interest of the restaurant. Fifteen million Americans suffer from some type of food allergy, and as allergy awareness continues to grow, restaurants are indeed paying attention. Restaurants are recognizing that not only is it important to be food allergy aware in general, but that by being accommodating to food allergy customers, they are welcoming a whole new population of customers who will increase their profit margin and promote the restaurant.[1]

So, what exactly are restaurants doing in order to protect those with food allergies? As of the publication of this book, only the states of Massachusetts and Rhode Island have legislation in place that mandates all restaurants go through some sort of food allergy and food sensitivity training, but it is likely that other states will follow suit.

The National Restaurant Association has made food allergy awareness and education a top priority for food allergic guests. It has partnered with FARE to create an online course for its restaurant staff to further their knowledge about how to provide a safe and great dining experience for those customers with food allergies.[2] The course has become integrated into the National Restaurant Association's promotion of food safety, touching on factors such as the eight major allergens, what cross-contamination is and how to prevent it, and open communication between the customer, the front-of-house staff, and the back-of-house staff. In fact, if you have been out to eat at a restaurant recently, you may have noticed that somewhere on the menu there is a sentence that may read something like "Please inform your server if someone in your party has a food allergy," which is a great way to begin the conversation. You may also notice that more and more menus also offer gluten-free options or even a separate menu for those who suffer from celiac disease, which is a step in the right direction and shows that a particular restaurant takes dietary needs seriously.

Show Your Appreciation

If you have gone out to eat and the restaurant staff seemed knowledgeable and understanding, and allowed you to have a pleasant dining experience, make sure that you let them know it is appreciated. Of course you can always give the wait-staff a good tip, but kind and positive words also go a long way. You can thank the server, manager, or chef directly, or simply speak to the manager on duty advising him or her how accommodating and wonderful the staff has been. Not only is this a thoughtful thing to do, but it also builds a good rapport with the staff and you will more likely be remembered each time you go out to eat at that restaurant. Appreciation can reinforce the steps that need to be taken in order for you to have a safe and fun experience. Additionally, you can go online and write positive reviews about the restaurant and staff, and one site in particular, www.allergyeats.com, is a great forum in which to do this.

The AllergyEats app was mentioned previously, but their website is also a great resource for anyone suffering from food allergies. AllergyEats was created

Allergy-Aware Chain Restaurants

According to feedback that AllergyEats received from its website and app, the following restaurant chains scored high with customers in 2014 for being food allergy aware and sensitive to the needs of customers with food allergies:

- Red Robin Gourmet Burgers
- P.F. Chang's China Bistro
- Chipotle Mexican Grill
- Outback Steakhouse
- Romano's Macaroni Grill
- Ninety-Nine Restaurant and Pub
- Uno Chicago Grill
- Bertucci's Brick Oven Pizzeria
- Papa Razzi Trattoria
- Legal Sea Foods
- Not Your Average Joe's[c]

"Special allergy menus do not work for me since I have multiple food allergies and not all of them are in the top eight. I need to be able to check all of the ingredients. If a restaurant does not have ingredients available then I cannot eat there. One other thing I always do, although it may seem obvious, is check my food before I eat it. For example, I am allergic to milk and one time while out to eat, I could see something yellow on the inside of my burger. At first I thought it was just mustard, but when I examined it, I realized it was cheese. Cheese had been removed from my burger, but small amounts remained. We spoke to the manager and asked for a new burger. We explained that everything that touches my food has to be clean and they were very nice about it."—Emily C.[d]

by a father of food allergic children and serves as a forum for those with food allergies to rate and review their own dining experiences. AllergyEats also hosts an annual conference for those within the restaurant industry and an annual ranking of the top chain restaurants that cater to those with food allergies.[3] This ranking is very good to know if you are someone who suffers from food allergies. If you are able to find a restaurant chain that is both accommodating and has a menu with ingredients that would be safe for you, it can make for a better experience. Having this information will also make you feel more comfortable if you are traveling. Chances are if you have already eaten at a chain restaurant safely, you will most likely be accommodated at any of that chain restaurant's locations.

However, always make sure to convey your food allergy needs to the server even if you have eaten at this same place time and time again. You have to remember that although you may have eaten safely at this chain restaurant before, there are still ingredients that you may be allergic to on the menu, and this needs to be stressed to the server who is helping you.

When all is said and done, it comes down to the communication among you, the server, and the chef—basically anyone who will be handling your food at a given moment in order for you to have a safe dining experience. Another important point to make is that if at any time you feel that you are not being understood with regard to your food allergies and how to keep safe, then simply do not eat at that restaurant. This is a universal rule at any restaurant you eat at whether it is in your hometown, throughout the nation, or on your international travels, which brings us to the next chapter in which we discuss being away from home in more depth.

It Happened to Me:
A Note from the Author Regarding Restaurants

Part of going out to eat at a restaurant is the social atmosphere that comes along with it. As long as you can communicate your needs you should be able to dine out safely. If you do not feel comfortable eating at the restaurant, as long as you would be OK to sit at the restaurant, do not miss out on an opportunity to socialize with friends. Of course you should not be expected to go out and sit at a restaurant while watching everyone else eat on a regular basis, but once in a while is OK.

Personally, when I was first diagnosed and still learning how to live with my allergies, I used to think that if I was not eating at the restaurant, then I just should not go. I was worried about being judged and what everyone would think of me not eating. I felt awkward, especially when I was constantly asked questions about my allergies throughout the entire time I was at the restaurant. Eventually, I realized that the reason people probably kept asking me questions was the fact that when I went out I already had the notion that I did not belong, which probably became evident in my body language and in my attitude without even realizing it. When I started feeling more comfortable and prepared to eat in advance if necessary, I actually found myself being able to relax and have a good time.

YOUR HOME AWAY FROM HOME

Just because you have food allergies, it does not mean that you have to forgo traveling nationally or even internationally. With the proper preparation and planning, you can travel on planes, trains, automobiles, or Vespas, and practically any other mode of transportation to any destination of your choosing. You do not have to be limited by your allergies, but you do have to take certain measures to ensure your safety while you are traveling. Since you are a teenager and not quite out on your own yet, more than likely you are traveling with your family. Although this can take any potential worries away from you because your immediate family will ultimately be responsible for you, it is important to start sharing in that responsibility. Additionally, now that you are getting older, and if your parents, grandparents, or caretakers allow it, you may plan an overnight trip with your friends. In particular, senior trips in high school are very common, and if your family tells you it is OK to go, it can be fun and a rite of passage that you should not miss because of your food allergies.

Do Your Research and Know before You Go

When it comes to traveling, the first thing that you need to do is research the area to which you are going. For instance, if you are planning a vacation, you most likely would not want to plan a trip to a remote location where there is little access to telephones and the nearest hospital would be a helicopter ride away. Wherever you decide to go, it is always a good idea to check out where the local emergency rooms are located and how far away the hospital would be in relation to where you are staying. It is also a good idea to check out where the closest pharmacies are in case you need to fill a prescription. Always remember to keep your doctor's number handy and even speak to your doctor about your travel plans. You could also ask your doctor if he or she has any recommendations for you. In addition, keep all of your auto-injector prescriptions up-to-date and take extra auto-injectors with you in case of an emergency. Taking extra auto-injectors with you is something to

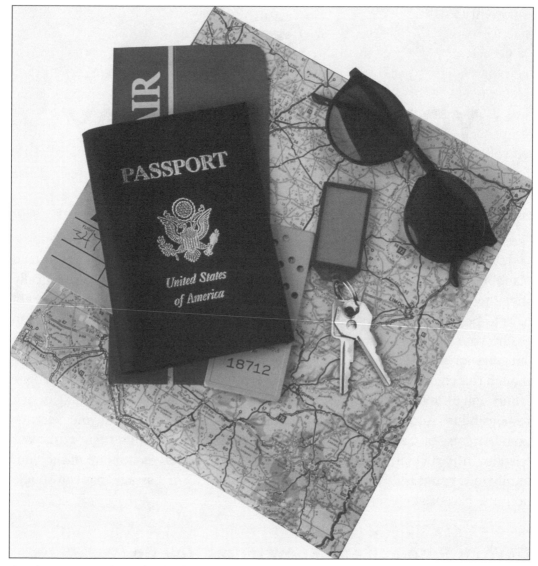

Just because you have food allergies does not mean you cannot travel.

discuss with your doctor as well. You may also need your parents, grandparents, or caretakers to contact your insurance company to check your coverage for extra prescriptions for the auto-injectors. Depending on what type of insurance you have, coverage may differ. However, some insurance companies have a provision for allowing an extra dose if you go on vacation.

Insurance Plans When It Comes to Traveling

Earlier we discussed insurance plans as they pertain to health care coverage with a primary care doctor and your allergist. However, the topic of insurance is also important to discuss when it comes to traveling. As you may be aware, insurance coverage can change every year, so it is important to know the plan that you have. Of course, if you or the insurance policyholder have any questions, then you or the policyholder should contact the health insurance company directly. Oftentimes the customer service number is right on the back of the health insurance card. Remember that prescription coverage is dictated by the health insurance company directly, and your allergist or primary care physician will not be able to tell you specific answers to your coverage questions. This is especially important if you are traveling abroad. Be sure to contact your health insurer to find out what type of coverage you have if you were to have an allergic reaction overseas, including, but not limited to, prescription coverage, emergency care, and both in-patient and out-patient coverage. It is important to note that even if you have coverage overseas, if you were to incur medical expenses while overseas, you may first have to pay out of pocket and be reimbursed by the insurance company once you are home. You will, of course, want to keep any and all receipts or copies of medical bills to submit to the insurance company for such reimbursement if it is necessary.

Travel Insurance

Additionally, while on the subject of insurance, it may be prudent for you or your family to purchase travel insurance in preparation for your vacation. Travel insurance will financially protect you in case you are not able to go on your vacation or if you cannot complete your vacation due to a medical emergency. It will also have provisions to financially protect you if your luggage is lost.[1] Many credit card companies such as American Express or business entities such as AAA have travel insurance or protection as part of their benefits, but there are also many private companies that offer travel insurance. Be sure to do research with your family to make sure that the companies you are looking into are reputable. When it comes to traveling abroad, for more information about travel insurance, travel precautions to take, or travel advisories, you can visit the U.S. Department of State's website at www.travel.state.gov.

There are other important things to remember while traveling, especially if traveling abroad. For example, always wear your medical identification bracelets, necklaces, and so on. Quite frankly, you should always wear medical identification, whether you are at home or away. You should also bring chef cards as mentioned earlier, and have those chef cards translated into the native language of the country you will be visiting, if you are traveling abroad. It would also be beneficial to carry a letter from your doctor that indicates your allergies and explains that he or she is your treating physician or allergist. Hopefully you will not run into any issues while traveling or while at your destination, but it is never a bad thing to be too prepared and have a good time than to be underprepared and risk having your vacation ruined. You want to plan for the worst-case scenario so that you reduce the risk of having an allergic reaction.

Choose the Right Accommodation

As part of your travel plans, not only is the choice of destination important, but the type of accommodation can be equally important. Depending on where you want to go and what type of vacation you or your family are planning, it may be a better idea to rent a place where there is a full kitchen, such as an apartment suite or a villa. This is actually very easy to do if you are traveling abroad. Many accommodations abroad have different types of villas for rent and can be just as luxurious as staying in a five-star hotel. Sometimes apartment suites or villas have special benefits, such as private beaches and docks, deals in local shops, or deals on a local tour. Another added benefit for someone suffering from food allergies is that with a kitchen, you have the added comfort of knowing that you can prepare your own food and snacks. You will have all of the control and none of the anxiety if you know that you have the option to cook your own food.

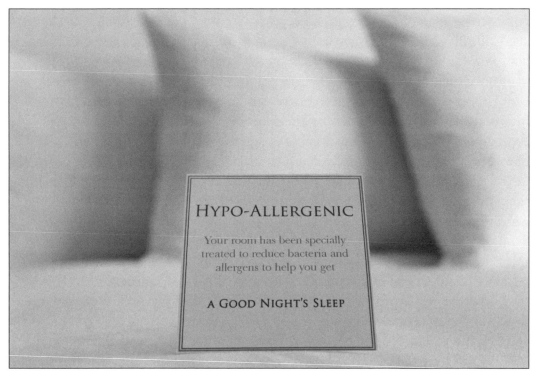

HYPO-ALLERGENIC

Your room has been specially treated to reduce bacteria and allergens to help you get

A GOOD NIGHT'S SLEEP

Many hotels now have allergy-friendly rooms. Be sure to always check accommodations so that they suit your needs.

Accommodating Hotel Chains

Some hotel chains that offer suites with a full kitchen or kitchenettes include

- Homewood Suites
- Embassy Suites
- DoubleTree
- Hyatt

Although these are chains that offer a full kitchen or kitchenette, always be sure to check with the individual hotel you will be staying at before booking to confirm.

Even if you do not stay at a place with a full-service kitchen, kitchenettes can be the next best thing. A great number of hotels in the United States now have certain rooms available that include kitchenettes. Sometimes, if the hotel room does not have a kitchenette and you are only planning on staying a night or two, you can inquire whether the hotel can put a mini-fridge in your room. You can also inquire if there is a microwave that you will be able to access. That way you can prepare a few meals ahead of time and freeze them to take with you on your journey. Of course, this will also depend on how far you are traveling. You will not want the safe prepared food to thaw and sit unrefrigerated for hours on end. Additionally, if you do stay in a hotel, it will be important to contact the hotel ahead of time to find out what its food policies are.

Hotels

As food allergies have become more well-known, restaurants, especially those within the hotel industry, have developed their own policies on how to handle customers with food allergies. This is also the case with staying at resorts. For instance, Disney World is one resort that works with its guests in trying to accommodate those with food allergies and dietary needs. If planning a trip to Disney World, contact Disney's special dietary needs department where you can find information about contacting the appropriate people, whether within the hotel where you are staying or within a Disney park itself, to best accommodate your allergy needs. Certain Disney parks also offer prepackaged allergy-friendly snacks for their guests from such companies as Enjoy Life Foods. Within certain parks, there are also kiosks available that can assist guests with food allergies in choosing restaurants, prepackaged snacks, and other allergy information.[2] Additionally, in 2014 Disney partnered with Mylan, makers of EpiPen, to provide stock epinephrine in all of its parks as well as on its cruise lines. In addition to providing these services, Disney now has trained nurses to administer the EpiPens at its first aid stations during normal business hours in case an emergency situation occurs. Together with Mylan, Disney will also offer educational resources to promote allergy awareness.[3]

Before going ahead and booking any hotel, whether at a resort or not, it is always a good idea to ask the staff at the hotel what its recommendations are for dining out with food allergies as well as options for other dining facilities. Once you have received recommendations, contact the recommended restaurant or dining facility to ask if it is equipped to handle your food allergies. In most cases, if you speak with the restaurant manager, he will be able to accommodate you to the best of his ability. If, after speaking with the restaurant manager, chef, or other staff, you feel comfortable and you do decide to eat at these restaurants, the same rules would apply as if you were eating at a restaurant close to home. Be sure to call ahead but be sure to keep safe snacks for you to eat just in case of an emergency. If the manager is not able to accommodate you, then contact the next restaurant on the list of referred places to eat. Again, the same rules apply as if you were eating at a restaurant close to home. If you cannot find a restaurant that will be able to accommodate you or if you do not feel confident that the manager or waitstaff understands your allergies, then simply do not eat at that restaurant.

Cruises

Now that we have discussed hotels, apartment suites, and villas, what do you do if you decide to go on a cruise? Of course, as with anything, make sure to do your research. Each individual cruise line will have its own policy on how to handle cruisers with special dietary needs, including those with food allergies. It will be essential for you to inquire about how the cruise line will accommodate guests with food allergies before booking the trip. At the time of booking you will also want to ask how medical emergencies are handled. All cruise lines are equipped to handle medical emergencies until they reach a port. Ask specifically how the cruise line handles an allergic reaction and anaphylactic attack. Be sure to ask if the cruise line carries epinephrine on board. Depending on the cruise line, you may also have to notify them in writing about your allergy or complete a special form indicating what your allergies are and what type of food is safe for you. This information will be given to the staff preparing and handling your food, but it is important to remind your waitstaff every time you eat. As a general rule, you will want to communicate your needs to the head waiter first and then speak to any waitstaff you will encounter thereafter. More than likely, you will have the same waitstaff for your lunch and dinner, and you can preorder your meals for the next day. Even if you do have the same waitstaff, be sure to remind them about your

Cruise Policies for Food Allergic Travelers

According to the Norwegian Cruise Line website, the company suggests that those travelers who have food allergies contact the access desk before booking to discuss policies and procedures in greater detail. Accommodations will vary depending on the country of destination of the cruise and the guest's particular allergy.[a]

Carnival Cruise Lines suggests on its website that it is able to accommodate those travelers with special dietary requests, including those with food allergies, if you speak to the dining team the first night of the cruise. These accommodations can be made in the main dining room only.[b] Although this is the suggested protocol on the cruise line's website, it would be a good idea to contact Carnival ahead of booking your trip to ensure that you will in fact be accommodated and that there will be little room for error.

Disney Cruise Line requires guests to complete a special form thirty days prior to departure. It also states that most food requests can be accommodated in table-service restaurants and that the head server must be notified of a guest's allergies.[c] However, it clearly states on the form that not all dietary requests can be honored, so it would be important to contact the cruise line prior to booking.

Royal Caribbean International advises on its website that guests should contact their travel planner, booking agent, or the Royal Caribbean itself to notify the cruise staff of a food allergy. Most food allergies can be accommodated, but the cruise line will need to know ninety days prior to departure for a European/South American Cruise and forty-five days prior to any other departure.[d]

food allergies each and every time you sit down to eat. More than likely, the same staff will remember you, but there can be thousands of people on a cruise ship at one time. Never assume that you only have to remind the staff about your allergies once. Even if they do remember you, they may not remember your specific allergies. It is a good idea to have your meals in the main dining room and avoid the buffets as the risk of cross-contamination can be extremely high.[4] Many people with food allergies have taken cruises without incident, but you want to be sure to go over all of the risks and policies with your family before making a decision. This is also true when you decide on which airline you will be flying in order to get to your vacation spot.

Flying

Flying can be an anxiety-producing experience for a lot of people who are claustrophobic or simply think of flying as being enclosed in a capsule thousands of feet in the air. For those who suffer from food allergies, being stuck in an enclosed capsule thousands of feet in the air with your allergen can seem like a great beginning to the script for a horror movie. It is important to remember that people with food allergies fly every day without incident. This means that you can travel safely by air, too; just make sure you take the necessary precautions.

Since airlines are all privately run, just like any individual hotel or resort you would be staying at, they have their own policies as to accommodating passengers with food allergies. Some policies are better than others. You can research individual airline policies by going to the airlines' websites as most have their policies available online. For instance, if you are allergic to peanuts or tree nuts, it is important to note that some airlines will serve peanuts or tree nuts as a snack on a regular basis. However, if told in advance, the steward would offer a peanut/tree-nut-free snack during your flight. Some airlines have a peanut-free policy where they do not serve peanuts at all, but they may serve a trail mix that contains tree nuts. Another important factor is that some airlines that state they will not serve peanuts or tree nuts as a snack may still serve nuts in their first-class section. Other airlines may have what they call a "buffer zone" where they will ask passengers sitting a few rows in front of you or behind you to refrain from eating nuts, creating a small buffer. It is important to note that just because an airline, or any facility where food is served for that matter, states that peanuts will not be served, it does not necessarily mean that the airline is completely nut free. Additionally, no airline can claim to be 100 percent peanut free or free from your particular allergen because it cannot control every food that passengers may bring on the flight. Depending on the airline and the crew, the crew may offer to make an announcement indicating that there is a passenger on board who has severe food allergies and ask that other passengers refrain from eating the offending food. However, this will be up to the crew.

In 2002, the Federal Aviation Administration (FAA) issued an advisory circular offering guidelines to crews and passengers on how to handle allergens in the air.[5] It is very important to note that these are simply guidelines and are not enforceable. As mentioned before, because airlines are privately owned and are not federally funded, the FAA and other government bodies do not govern each individual airline's policy. While every airline is free to make its own rules and policies while in the air, the 1986 Air Carrier Access Act, which is enforceable by the U.S. Department of Transportation, does provide some assistance to individuals who have physical or mental impairments. Included in part 382 of this act, epinephrine is required to be on board an aircraft. However, if a medical emergency were to occur in flight, airline policy dictates that, although flight attendants have first-aid training, they cannot administer any medications or emergency assistance unless there is a board-certified doctor on the flight or medical services have been radioed on the ground first. Additionally, it is also important to note that if the airplane has to make an emergency landing, this action will be at the sole discretion of the pilot.[6] Clearly, this policy needs fine-tuning. If there is a medical emergency and the flight attendants have been medically trained, they should not need to ask permission to save someone's life or help someone. What it does illustrate, however, is the fact that behind any policy, behind any guideline are people. People make up the crew. People need to communicate with you about your allergies, and these people will have to decide to take on the responsibility to assist you in reducing your risk of having an allergic reaction.

For instance, say you are traveling from the East Coast of the United States to the West Coast, and you have a layover on the way to your ultimate destination. You have spoken with the reservation agent about your allergies, reminded the worker at the gate about your allergies, and then proceeded to tell the crew on board about your allergies, who assure you that they have created a buffer zone for you and that no nut snacks will be served on the flight. Once you are in the air, snacks are being served and you notice that there are bags of trail mix, which contain nuts, for sale. When you ask that the bags not be served because you had been told that there will be no nuts in the snacks, the flight attendant takes out a manual and says that there are no peanuts in the trail mix. The attendant has to serve them because she must give each passenger at least three different choices of snacks according to the manual. She is mistaken on the no nuts being served at all, but there is nothing she can do at this point because, after all, the manual states the policy. A fellow passenger who ordered the trail mix overhears the conversation and gives it back to the flight attendant and states that two choices of snacks would be just fine if it means that you will not have an allergic reaction, and the other passengers follow suit. You thank your fellow passengers and sit anxiously until your next leg of the journey, dreading when you have to switch crews after your layover and worrying you will have to go through this ordeal again. However, when the time comes to inform the second crew, it is like you are dealing with a completely different airline. You are not made to feel like an inconvenience; you are taken care of. Not only do you have a wonderful flight, but your faith in humanity is now restored.

Believe it or not, the previous scenario was actually a true experience of mine and shows how important it is to always communicate your needs because help will come from somewhere. Although the flight attendant did not offer assistance, fellow passengers stepped up to the plate, and the crew on the second leg of the journey could not have been more accommodating. Although you may feel that your safety when it comes to not having an allergic reaction is at the discretion of others, there are steps you can take to reduce your risk of having a reaction while on a plane. One of the most important things to remember is that people suffering from food allergies fly all of the time without a problem. You can too!

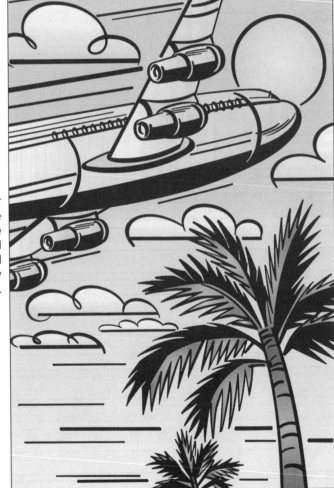

Airline travel can be scary for those with food allergies. Be sure to always check airline policies before you fly, and remember that people with food allergies fly safely every day with the proper precautions.

Airline Policies for Those with Nut Allergies

American Airlines does not serve peanuts, but it does serve tree nuts as part of its snacks. American Airlines specifically states on its website that it "[does] not have in place procedures that allow flight crews to not serve these foods upon request of the customer" and that it "will not provide nut buffer zones." Although the planes are cleaned regularly, American Airlines cannot guarantee that residue will be completely removed from the plane or that other customers will not bring nut products on board.[e]

Delta Air Lines suggests on its website to contact Delta sales support or reservations to note that a passenger has a nut allergy. The company also suggests that it will serve nonpeanut products during the flight and offer nut allergic passengers the opportunity to preboard to clean the seating area as needed.[f]

JetBlue does not serve any peanut products on its flights, but cannot guarantee what other passengers will bring on board. For that reason, if informed that a passenger has a nut allergy, JetBlue will create a buffer zone for that passenger. Additionally, JetBlue offers many nonnut snacks, including the peanut- and tree-nut-free Chocolate Chip Minis cookies from Skeeter Snacks.[g]

Southwest Airlines does serve peanuts, but it will serve alternative snacks if made aware that a passenger has a nut allergy. The airline suggests that all passengers with a nut allergy call to book their flights rather than book online and to try to book a flight earlier in the morning if at all possible to minimize the risk of contamination. Southwest also requires passengers who have a nut allergy to arrive at least one hour before departure time to clean down the seating area and reconfirm allergy with appropriate crew.[h]

United Airlines does not serve prepackaged peanuts, but it does serve other nut snacks and snacks that may be cross-contaminated with peanut. The crew may be notified that you suffer from a nut allergy, but United will not offer buffer zones and will not remove onboard products based on passenger concerns.[i]

1. First and foremost, look up the airline's allergy policy online.
2. Contact the airline over the phone and speak to a reservation agent directly to discuss your allergies and allergy accommodations that can be made for you.
3. Discuss your travel plans with your doctor, making sure to get a refill on your auto-injectors and/or take extra if needed, as well as a note stating your allergies with your doctor's contact information. Be sure to save the original prescription package when traveling and keep it with you for easy access on the flight.
4. Prepare and pack safe foods to bring with you during the flight. Although some airlines offer special dietary meals it would not be wise to eat any airline food because of the risk of cross-contamination.
5. Be sure to wipe down the seats and tray tables before sitting as they can contain residue from previous passengers. Bring a seat cover and your own pillow or blankets. Do not use the ones from the airlines as they, too, can

It Happened to Me:

A Note from the Author Regarding International Travel

My brother and sister are world travelers, but I, on the other hand, never travel too far from home. Part of the reason for this is that once I was diagnosed with food allergies, I was not only afraid of flying, but I was afraid of traveling to any destination I was not familiar with. However, when my husband and I decided to get married, we knew that we wanted to go somewhere for our honeymoon that we would always remember. It was decided that we would travel to the south of Italy in Ravello, then go by train to Florence, and then to Rome. We would be staying at villas the entire time, which all had kitchens; that way I would be able to cook everything myself, just like I would have done if we were to go somewhere in the United States or even in my own home. I also made sure that there were doctors and hospitals near each place we were staying and discussed all of my travel plans with my doctor. I would bring more than enough auto-injectors in case anything happened, and I also would pack a suitcase of foods that I knew would be safe in case it took a while to get to where we needed to be. It was such a worthwhile trip. I was so glad that I could put my fear aside and enjoy the moment. With enough preparations and knowledge, you can travel anywhere, too!

contain residue of your allergens. If at all possible, try to book an early flight to minimize the risk of residue and other allergens.

College—Your Home Away from Home

Now that we have discussed traveling in terms of accommodations, traveling by land, and traveling by sea, probably the next most important home away from home that you will experience is going off to college. If you do choose to go to college, there are quite a few decisions to make before you go. Do you have a specific subject area that you would like to study? If so, then you may want to target your search to a school specializing in that area. Do you want to go to a large school or a small school? Do you want to go to school in a suburb or in a large metropolitan city? Do you want to be paying off your student loans for thirty years after you graduate or go to a school that is more affordable? Do you want to live at school or commute from home? These are just some of the factors that need to be considered when choosing a college. However, if you have food allergies, there are a few more factors that you will need to consider, such as will the school make accommodations for you because of your allergies? How will you deal with a roommate? Should you live in a single? Would it be more beneficial to you to have an apartment with a fully working kitchen so you can make your own meals, or should you go with the school's meal plan as is? Not to worry; allergies are becoming more common and more well-known throughout colleges and universities. The issue of food allergies and accommodations at colleges and universities may have become even more well-known as a result of a settlement between Lesley University and the U.S. Justice Department in December of 2012.

If you are not familiar with this settlement, students who lived on campus at Lesley University in Cambridge, Massachusetts, lodged a complaint with the Justice Department stating that the university violated the Americans with Disabilities Act. These students alleged that their rights were being violated due to the fact that they were being forced to pay for a meal plan that made no accommodations for their special dietary needs, whether it be food allergies or celiac disease. In fact, some of the students had such severe food allergies that they never even used the dining services at all. Under the settlement, Lesley University agreed to a number of terms to accommodate the current students as well as any future students, but particularly the following provisions:

- Provide gluten-free and allergen-free food options in its dining hall food lines in addition to its standard meal options
- Allow students with known allergies to preorder allergen-free meals
- Display notices concerning food allergies and identify foods containing specific allergens

- Train food service and university staff about food allergy-related issues
- Provide a dedicated space in its main dining hall to store and prepare gluten-free and allergen-free foods
- Work to retain vendors that accept students' prepaid meal cards that also offer food without allergens[7]

This agreement not only was a tremendously positive outcome for the students at Lesley University who lodged the complaint, but it also served as a great model for other schools across the country on how best to accommodate those students with food allergies, celiac disease, and other dietary needs. Now it is quite common and even expected that most colleges and universities will be able to accommodate you as long as you take the first step in informing the school about your need for a special dietary accommodation.

When I spoke with Kimberly Pierce, RD, LDN, and Sodexo dietitian at Stonehill College in Easton, Massachusetts, she advised that there are very few situations in which the dining services team could not accommodate a student who suffers from food allergies. As Ms. Pierce noted, an important part of eating is the social experience,[8] and this is true about college in general: it is much more than the academic experience; it is a social experience as well. You should not be restricted in your experiences just because of your food allergies.

Ms. Pierce went on to explain that prospective students should first look on the website of the school that interests them and search around the dining services area of the website. The prospective student should seek out the e-mail or other contact information for either the registered dietitian the school has on staff or the person in charge of dining services. The prospective student should get in touch with that person to discuss how the school is equipped to handle food allergies. If the school looks promising, then a campus tour could be scheduled, making sure to include a tour of the dining commons and to schedule a meeting with the head chef.[9]

After much deliberation and contemplation, when you finally choose a school to attend, you will be asked to complete a health form, where you will list your allergies. However, Ms. Pierce made an important point *that because of privacy regulations, your health information goes directly to medical services. It is not shared with any other part of the school unless you take the initiative to allow it to be shared.*

> "I have found that the chef and those in charge of managing the dining hall on campuses are the most informed and very helpful people who are familiar with food allergies, ingredients, and safe practices."—Ryan M.[j]

If you do not contact dining services or someone from the kitchen staff, then there is no way for them to know about your allergies.[10] With that being said, if you do decide to live on campus, it is also important to contact the office of disabilities as well as the residence life staff to determine how your allergies will be handled in the dormitories and by any potential roommates.[11] In case you are not familiar with the residence life staff and what their roles are at college—they are people who ensure that your transition to living on campus is a smooth one. They help to create a community and positive living environment for those who do choose to live on campus. They also ensure that those living on campus uphold the rules of the school and are respectful to other students and roommates.

The idea of sharing a room with a complete stranger can seem somewhat daunting, especially if you have food allergies. You may be wondering what your roommate will think and worried that he or she may like the very foods you are allergic to. This is an important reason why you need to contact the school's residence life staff as well as the office of disabilities. You need to understand the school's policies and how the school and school staff will be able to accommodate you in terms of selecting an appropriate room and roommate. In general, you will be asked to fill out a questionnaire so that the school can match you up with someone who has similar habits as you. This form is also a good place to note your allergies.

Roommate assignments are given well in advance of the official move-in date, so it is strongly suggested that you contact your potential roommate to discuss how you will be living together. This is the time to inform your potential roommate about the seriousness of your food allergies. As with anyone new to whom you are explaining your allergies, you will need to go over what allergies are, your particular symptoms, where your auto-injectors are stored, and how to administer your auto-injector in case of an emergency. You need to discuss the possibility that your roommate not bring the offending food into the room at all. Many college students with food allergies have successfully had this talk with their roommates and continue to live amicably and easily together. However, you do have to be aware that for someone who is not used to sharing a room with another person in such close quarters coupled with accommodating you in regard to your food allergies, it may be too much to handle. Do not lose heart. It is better to know that this would not be a good living situation before it begins. If you are aware of this early on, you can contact residence life to get a new roommate assignment. There are a lot of adjustments that you will be making as you enter into college, and anything you can do to avoid potential issues should be welcomed and taken advantage of.[12] Once you make all of your necessary contacts regarding your potential home away from home, you will find that there are many resources available to you. Additionally, once everyone who will be involved with keeping you safe is made aware of your food allergies, you will be followed and monitored throughout your college career.

As a general rule, the registered dietitian or the head of dining services will first have a meeting with you to learn exactly what you are allergic to and how the menu can be altered in order to accommodate you. Depending on the severity of your food allergies, accommodations will need to be made on a case-by-case basis, of course. It is good to have regular meetings with the chef and registered dietitian to stay current on menu items and to keep the risk of cross-contamination to a minimum. Also, depending on the size of the school and the student body and the kitchen services, you might have other options. For example, if the school is small, then you may be able to call in your meals ahead of time. The dining staff may be able to put in a special order for you that can be relayed to the server or other kitchen staff when you pick up your food. Since you will have a set schedule each semester, by calling ahead, you can coordinate the times that you will need to eat breakfast, lunch, and dinner. If this turns out to be an option at your particular school, when you pick up your food, always make sure to remind the servers to double-check with the chef to ensure that the meal is allergy friendly for you. Many times, the meals will be planned well in advance and you can go over menu items with the registered dietitian, chef, and/or head of dining services. If you are vocal about your allergies and attend the regular meetings, you will become familiar with not only the chefs who are cooking your food, but the rest of the dining staff serving the food as well. If you build a rapport with all of the staff it will decrease your chances of your message getting lost in translation, so to speak, and everyone will be on the same page when it comes to keeping you safe.

Another important point to consider is that you will most definitely not be the only one suffering from food allergies. You will have fellow classmates who suffer from them as well. Get to know these classmates. You may even find that there are already groups on campus that are devoted to food allergies and food sensitivities. If there is not a group already on campus, think about starting one yourself, just like Mackenzie, age nineteen, did at her college.

I have just started a club on campus called the Food Allergy Awareness Club! A lot of people signed up at the club fair. The purpose of the club is to advocate for those with specific dietary needs, serve as a support group, and create a safe and inclusive atmosphere in the dorms and dining halls. Students without dietary restrictions are also welcome! Our goal is to spread knowledge and understanding of the growing epidemic of food allergies. My motto is: "Together we can find solutions." I hope to work with dining services and increase options in the dining halls for people with allergies. I am thrilled there are options even to begin with, but I think we can improve!

Before I even applied to a school, I called ahead, gave them the low down, and instantly knew if I would be safe there. If the college wasn't confident in being able to keep me safe, I sure as heck wasn't going to spend 4 years there eating ramen! And my parents weren't going to pay for me not to eat. They have to be able to sleep at night. So, I was only allowed to look at colleges in the northeast, because if something happened, my parents didn't want to have to catch a flight. When I called the current college I am attending now, they were very assuring, and I was overjoyed by the fact that they had a food station that completely eliminated the eight top allergens from its cooking facility!! I eat there every day.

Mackenzie is also a Teen Advisor with FARE (Food Allergy Education & Research) and had this to say about her role as an advisor and her wish to continue to spread food allergy awareness and education:

I really wanted to help let kids with food allergies know that they're not alone. We can all get through this together and learn from each other's experiences—good and bad. The people in my generation are the pioneers for food allergy awareness. This is a new and growing epidemic. If we don't make change, no one will! So being a Teen Advisor allows me to connect with other kids and young adults who want to make change. Remember the ABCs of allergy awareness: Advocacy Builds Confidence. (I came up with that when I was creating my club.) YOU are your only advocate, and you can't be afraid to stand up for yourself. ANY chance you have to educate others, take advantage of it! Sooner or later, it won't be such a foreign concept, and we can feel more safe and included.[13]

You are continually working on creating your own world while exploring the world around you and part of this exploration is being aware of what is going into and on your body. Knowing the importance of reading each and every ingredient label is extremely important and will be the topic discussed in the next chapter.

THE IMPORTANCE OF READING LABELS

Somewhere along your journey into middle school or high school, you may have been required to take a foreign language. If learning new languages was, or is, a requirement for your education, then you undoubtedly have picked up some understanding of them. Reading ingredient labels on food and food products is much like learning a foreign language. Sometimes it may seem that the ingredients themselves are written in a foreign language with words such as *hydrolyzed protein*, *casein*, *whey*, and so on, although that is not the case. While it may seem difficult to go through a paragraph of ingredients every time you wish to purchase food, once you get the hang of it and know what to look for when reading a label, it will automatically become part of your routine. Reading labels is not just important for learning about food products that you are ingesting, but it is also important for learning about any substance that may go on your body, such as products for your personal hygiene like shampoos, soaps, makeup, and lotion. Whether you suffer from food allergies or not, it is important to know what goes in and on our bodies. This chapter will help you decipher some of the names that can be used in place of more commonly known names for certain allergens and explain what to look for when you are reading an ingredient label.

You may have seen television commercials for food-related products boasting that the manufacturers of these products only use all-natural ingredients or certain drink products which contain nothing less than 100 percent juice. These companies seem to be very proud of the fact that they are using all-natural ingredients, which may have you asking the larger question of why? Shouldn't all of the food or drinks we ingest be all natural? Should we expect anything less of our food than the actual food itself? The truth of the matter is, a majority of people do not pay attention to the ingredients in their food because they have not had a reason to do so. If you suffer from food allergies, you always need to pay attention to ingredients in foods and this is a good thing. Everyone, whether food allergic or not, should be paying attention to what is considered "food." If you suffer from food allergies, you may have heard of a theory that one of the possible causes of the rise in food allergies has to do with artificial and genetically

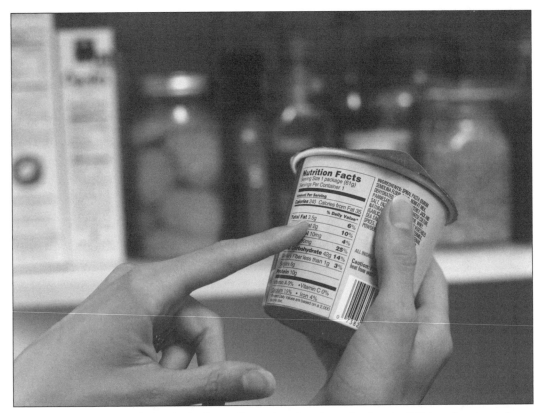

Always read labels and check the ingredients in a food product even if it is a food you have eaten before.

modified ingredients in food that were never present in earlier generations. Although this is just a theory and there is little to no scientific evidence to support this claim, it does make one pause to consider the possibility. Whether the claim is potentially true or not, there is a universal truth that making smart choices about what to eat and paying attention to the ingredients that are being used in the food your body takes in can have long-lasting benefits as you get older.

Just as it is vitally important to know what ingredients are going into your body, it is essential to be aware of how a label should be read to interpret such vital information.[1] In order to properly read labels, you must understand the food allergy labeling law enforced by the U.S. Food and Drug Administration (FDA).[2] The Food Allergen Labeling and Consumer Protection Act was passed in 2004 (Public Law 108-282, Title II) and ensures that all foods packaged after January 1, 2006, must declare in plain language whether they contain a protein from one of the eight major allergens (milk, egg, soy, peanuts, tree nuts, wheat, fish, and shellfish). If you were to look at an ingredient label, you might see the food allergen in parentheses in bold after a particular ingredient. Ingredients can also be listed within the body of the complete list of ingredients. At the bottom of the label, you may notice the word *contains* in bold with a list of the eight major allergens, if applicable. While this labeling law has made it much easier for those with food allergies to figure out if a packaged food contains a specific ingredient that they are allergic to, this is not a fool-proof way to avoid allergens or to be sure that the foods are 100 percent safe to eat for those people who suffer from multiple food allergies. The number one issue with the labeling law is that only proteins from the eight major allergens are required to be listed. If you are a person who suffers from a sesame seed allergy, for instance, there is no requirement for it to be listed and you would have to look over all of the ingredients to make sure that sesame seeds are not contained in the product. In addition, shellfish from the eight major allergens pertains to crustacean shellfish such as shrimp, crab, and lobster, and not shellfish from the mollusk family. If you are allergic to mussels, clams, or oysters, this may not be listed appropriately in the ingredient label. Also, raw fruits and vegetables along with refined oils (even if these oils come from one of the major allergens) and meat, poultry, or eggs do not need to be listed under this law. Additionally, there are no formal guidelines on the "May contain" statements beneath the actual "Contains" statement.[3]

Depending on the manufacturer, the "May contain" statement can include one of the eight allergens or you may also see "Processed on shared equipment" (with one of the major allergens). However, manufacturers are not required to have a "May contain" statement, although this should be worked into the labeling law as it can be helpful for people who are highly sensitive to allergic reactions. Even though the direct product may not contain one of the eight major allergens, there may be the teeniest, tiniest amount from shared equipment and albeit small, there may still be a risk of cross-contamination. If you are highly sensitive, then be sure to discuss this with your allergist in order to determine whether you should stay away from products that include the "Processed on shared equipment" or "May contain" language.

For the most part, the "May contain" language is helpful for those suffering from food allergies, but there have also been claims from some people in the food allergy community that certain companies and manufacturers have used the "May contain" language to declare the possibilities of the major allergens unnecessarily in order to minimize costs on actually determining whether the allergen is indeed in the food. If true, then this would be unfortunate for certain people staying away from products and food if in all actuality these people did not need to. However, a good rule of thumb is that if you ever have a question or doubt about certain ingredients or the way that something is packaged, then contact the manufacturer directly and discuss your concerns with your allergist. This is especially helpful if you have been eating one brand of food and notice that this manufacturer now produces a line with your allergen in it. It would be prudent to contact the manufacturer to find out if the new product and the product you have been eating will be processed in different facilities or, if in the same facility, if they will be produced on shared equipment. As someone who suffers from food allergies, you already have a modified diet or need to limit your diet in some manner, so it is foolish and inconvenient for you to put limitations on yourself to food or food products unnecessarily.

Never be afraid to ask questions or find out more information if you do not have enough knowledge on your own, and never assume that ingredients remain the same. Even if you have eaten a product ninety-nine times and the ingredients have not changed, the hundredth time could be the change and you need to be aware of it. If you have been reading labels and dealing with allergies for a while, you may have noticed that certain ingredients could be interchangeable in your favorite products, and one of those you may be allergic to while the other you are not. Additionally, if a product is labeled as having "natural flavor," "natural color," or "spice," those items do not have to be listed individually if they do not contain one of the top major allergens.[4] This may be confusing because you may be allergic to certain spices, but not all. If the label says "spice" but the specific spices are not listed individually on the ingredient label, it is best to avoid the food altogether. Always, always, always read the ingredient label, and as mentioned before, this not only applies to food or food products, but hygiene products as well.

Not only can food ingredients be in food, but they can also be found in other things such as animal food or bedding as well as personal hygiene items such as hair products, body products, makeup, and soap. Oftentimes with these types of products, it can be a little more difficult to determine if an allergen is present. You will have to look at the label in its entirety, although you should always look at a label in its entirety and not just the "Contains" statement in bold at the bottom of the ingredient list. Sometimes an allergen could be present, but it may be in such a long list of ingredients that it is hard to find. Do not skim over the ingredients. Read them every time and two or three times if need be.

Even though most of the products will not be ingested and just go onto your body, if you are highly sensitive and are at risk of having an allergic reaction, although not an anaphylactic reaction, why have the potential to be uncomfortable? For instance, if you go down the shampoo and conditioner aisle in your local store, you may notice common ingredients. A major ingredient in any brand is typically *hydrolyzed wheat protein* or *hydrolyzed soy protein*. If you have an allergy to wheat or to soy, this could pose a problem for you. Additionally, many hair products have plant extracts or oils derived from nuts.

Another point to remember is that while some hygiene products do contain certain man-made cleaning agents with very hard-to-pronounce names, many of them contain all-natural ingredients. However, ingredients such as nuts, soy, and wheat *are* natural, so just because a product is all natural, it does not mean that it is free from allergens. The same thing holds true if a product is labeled "hypoallergenic."

It Happened to Me:
A Note from the Author Regarding Labels

While in a night class that had just begun, with people I didn't get a chance to know yet, I was eating a snack that had no nuts or soy or any of the foods I am allergic to. No biggie, right? Wrong. I was eating my snack as I had for months when my throat started feeling funny. I remember thinking that there was no way I was allergic to this snack because it had always been safe for me. The truth is I had stopped reading the ingredients label after I realized it was safe for me to eat. I figured I was probably just getting nervous because it was a new class (actually I prayed that was the feeling I was having, but I knew better). I quickly took a drink, and the drink would not go down easily because my throat was swelling. I left the class and told the secretary that I needed to go to the hospital because I was having an allergic reaction.

I'm not very proud of the following, but I will share my stupidity so that you will not make the same mistake. Not only did I not use my auto-injector right away when I knew I was having an allergic reaction, but I jumped into a taxi and headed to the hospital. I flat out refused an ambulance, actually believing that a taxi would get me to the hospital faster. Not only was it stupid on my part, but I scared the poor secretary and taxi driver half to death in the process. I also lost out on twenty dollars because that was all I had in my bag for a ride that should have cost around seven or eight dollars. What was I thinking? At the time it made perfect sense to me, but looking back on the incident I cannot believe that I lost my judgment like that.

As soon as I got to the emergency room, they took me right away. I told them that my throat was swollen, but obviously I could still breathe and talk, although it was getting difficult, and that I hadn't taken my EpiPen. They hooked me up to a heart monitor and started an IV, but I realized I should probably call someone to let them know where I was and I started panicking. The nurse told me not to worry. They would work on getting me better; I should worry about myself and then I could call anyone I wanted. I disagreed, but there wasn't much I could do. I kept saying, "But I could die and nobody knows where I am. I didn't tell the school what hospital I was going to. I jumped in a taxi!" I didn't get very far though because I suddenly got this horrible feeling in my left arm and it was getting cold. I then realized that without even knowing it, I had been alternately making a fist and opening it for a while because I was losing circulation. I informed the nurse and was horrified when my arm suddenly looked like something out of the sci-fi channel. I was ready for an alien to burst out of my vein. The nurse quickly took the IV out and administered it in a different part of my arm. Then another nurse held up a huge needle and asked if I was allergic to Benadryl, advising me that most people weren't allergic to Benadryl, but there are some people who are and she didn't want me to have another reaction. I blurted out that I didn't know in between breaths, because they were getting shorter and shorter. "I guess there's only one way to find out," I heard her mumble, and in a matter of seconds, I started getting tunnel vision. My chest felt like I had five hundred tons of bricks on it and the pressure was increasing. I remember trying to cry out in pain, but there didn't seem to be enough air. Either that or it was being muffled by the beeping of the heart monitor, which went from 90 to 150 in a matter of a few seconds or less. My next thought was that it was ironic because I really thought I was going to die and nobody knew where I was. All of a sudden I felt someone grab my hand and an emergency room resident, who was around my age, started talking to me and told me just to look at him and my heart rate would go down. Give that resident a gold star because it worked! As he continued to make small talk to distract me, my heart rate was going down on its own. I got the okay to call my boyfriend, who appeared by my side in lightning speed.

It was a terrifying experience for me that quite possibly could have been completely averted if I had remembered or thought to read the labels on the snack I was eating in my night class. Upon further inspection and an inquiry to the manufacturer, I discovered that my safe food was no longer safe for me and was now processed on shared equipment. In fact, the labeling had changed shortly after I had first discovered that the snack would be safe for me. If I had continuously checked the label, then I would have known this fact. The lesson here is to *always* read ingredient labels no matter how many times you have previously eaten the food.

The term *hypoallergenic* is used by many manufacturers, specifically those who produce face lotions, soaps, and cosmetics, to describe their products' gentleness on the skin. These companies claim that the ingredients in their products are more soothing on the skin, which in turn will lead to fewer allergic reactions. These claims may in fact be true, but there is no actual scientific evidence supporting such claims. According to a 1978 *FDA Consumer* magazine article, the federal court "struck down an FDA regulation requiring cosmetic manufacturers to conduct tests to back up any claim that a product is 'hypoallergenic.'"[5] In

Tree Nut Scientific Names

The following is a list of various tree nuts and their scientific names compiled by the FDA. It is by no means a comprehensive list, but will most assuredly give you a better idea of what to be on the lookout for when you are reading ingredients related to tree nuts.

Almond—prunus dulcis

Beech nut—fagus spp.

Brazil nut—bertholletia excels

Butternut—juglans cinerea

Cashew—anacardium occidentale

Chestnut—castanea, or castanea pumila

Filbert/hazelnut—corylus spp.

Ginko nut—ginkgo biloba l.

Hickory Nut—carya spp.

Lichee nut—litchi chinensis sonn.

Macadamia nut/bush nut—macadamia spp.

Pecan—carya illinoensis

Pine nut—pinus spp.

Pili nut—canarium ovatum

Pistacio—pistacia vera l.

Sheanut—vitellaria paradoxa

Walnut—juglans[a]

simple terms, this means that any company can claim that its product or products are hypoallergenic or allergy tested. Maybe these companies do in fact go through extensive testing regarding allergies or the harshness of their products on the skin. Without any concrete hypoallergenic regulations or a governing body such as the FDA to create and to enforce regulations if they exist, this is a baseless claim. No merit can be given to a product simply based on advertising that it is hypoallergenic.

The bottom line: always read the list of ingredients. If you cannot pronounce an ingredient or if you have any question in your mind, then do not use that product or eat the food. Sometimes an answer to your question can be found by simply contacting the manufacturer. It is also helpful to learn the scientific names or other common names of the foods that you are allergic to, to give you one more level of awareness that may assist you when reading ingredient labels. For instance, if you see the ingredient *maltodextrin* or *maize*, these are terms that can be used for corn. If you see the ingredients *casein* or *whey*, these are proteins that are found in milk. If you see the term *albumin*, this is a protein found in egg. As for scientific names, peanuts are also known as arachis hypogea l.[6] You may see arachis oil in some cosmetic products or soaps or lotions. This is really peanut oil, so be aware!

Additionally, it is not only important to familiarize yourself with ingredients along with common and scientific names, but it is also important to familiarize yourself with dishes or entrées that may contain these ingredients. For instance, pesto sauce typically comes with pine nuts mixed into it, although you may not be able to see the actual nuts in the dish. If you were to go out to a restaurant or if you were picking up a jar of pesto sauce, pine nuts would be an important ingredient to look for, possibly by their scientific name, and more than likely you should avoid pesto sauce altogether if you have a tree nut allergy. Additionally, some pastries and breads have an egg wash on them that is not necessarily listed as part of the ingredients.

Knowing what ingredients go into certain dishes and having the ability to cook for yourself are important skills for anyone, but it is even more important if you are someone who suffers from food allergies. This topic will be explored in greater depth in the next chapter.

TOP CHEF: COOKING WELL AND LIVING WELL WITH DIETARY RESTRICTIONS

N ow that you have explored different ways to deal with your food allergies and how to deal with your allergies in different settings, you should be feeling more empowered and more in control. This is an important step in becoming independent and learning to continually self-advocate. With that being said, it is time to take it a step further. Now it is time to get your hands messy! Are you ready? It is time to learn how to cook and how to plan meals for less stress as you get older. If you have an interest in cooking already, that is wonderful! If there are twenty-five things that you would rather be doing and cooking is on the bottom of your list, then that is OK, too. Regardless of where you fall on your cooking preference level, if you have food allergies, you will need to learn how to do some cooking for yourself.

As someone who suffers from food allergies, you should have an arsenal of safe foods and go-to meals that you can prepare in case of travel, last-minute outings, or events, or to have handy in case a preplanned meal at a party or a restaurant does not work out. As mentioned in earlier chapters, your parents, grandparents, or caretakers have probably been the ones who prepare most of your meals, including doing the shopping that goes along with obtaining allergy-safe ingredients. These family members will not be with you at every meal, especially if you are planning on going away to college or are ready to move out on your own in a few years, so you need to learn how to cook for yourself. Do not view cooking with regard to your food allergies as a chore; rather, look at it as another way to be more creative in the kitchen with new discoveries to be made. You can learn to become a great chef as well as a detective and a scientist. Look for safe ingredients, figure out which ingredients are used to make a desired chemical reaction in order

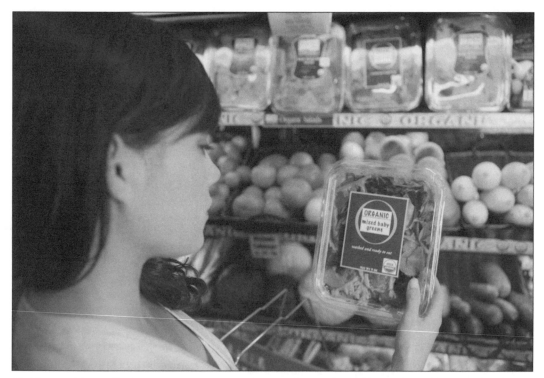

Picking out ingredients gets easier as you learn what to look for, and cooking can be fun!

to create the food, and figure out a food you can have to substitute in that chemical reaction without sacrificing taste. Cooking can be exciting and a lot of fun!

Prepare Your Kitchen

In the previous chapter you learned how to read ingredient labels, which is one of the major steps you will need to learn in order to prepare your own meals. Another important factor in learning to cook for yourself, especially if you are living in a household with people who do not suffer from food allergies, is how to set up the kitchen. Now, you do not have to completely redesign a kitchen and rethink the way you prepare food, but there are certain steps you can take in order to minimize cross-contamination.

First, and probably the easiest thing you can do, is to designate certain shelves or even an entire cabinet to the allergy-friendly foods you can eat. This way, your food is all in one spot and there will be very little risk of getting residue from an allergen onto the boxes of food or food products that you can eat. The next thing you can do is to put labels on your boxes of food or food products to ensure that extra level of safety. You could also choose to label Tupperware or other containers or even get a different color of Tupperware, glassware, or silverware to make it that much easier to determine which ones are safe for you. Additionally, it may

Label It!

For some great allergy labels, check out Mabel's Labels (www.mabelslabels. com/products/Allergy-Alert-Labels/), which has customizable food allergy labels that make it easy to distinguish between those food items or containers that contain allergy-friendly foods and those that do not.

be a good idea to have separate cooking utensils such as tongs, spoons, or ladles. A definite must-do is to have different sponges and/or cleaning pads for your dishes, utensils, and so on. That way there is no chance of getting residue from an allergen transferred from a dirty dish to a sponge/cleaning utensil to your dish or utensil. Once you have a properly organized kitchen, you are on your way to becoming an expert chef!

Ingredient Substitutions

In the previous chapter, you learned how to read ingredients, but now it will be important to learn which ingredients you may be able to completely omit from a recipe or which foods you can use as a substitute for the ingredients you are allergic to. This is when you can really become a detective and where cooking can become a science. If a recipe can still work by leaving a certain ingredient out, then no problem. Sometimes, especially if you are baking, ingredients play a role in creating some sort of reaction with the other ingredients to provide the desired effect, or in this case, the desired meal or dessert. Most baked goods contain eggs, which are used to keep the food together or to help the food to rise. In some recipes, you can substitute one quarter cup of applesauce, banana, or other pureed fruit for every one egg that the recipe calls for in order to create the same effect. You can also use a product called xantham gum as an egg replacer. If you do use an egg replacer, be careful not to confuse it with an egg substitute. Egg substitutes still contain egg and are re-formularized for people concerned about their cholesterol, not for those people with food allergies to egg. As with any product, you will need to make sure to read all the ingredients on any substitution product you buy, looking to make sure that it is not processed in a facility that produces other foods that you may be allergic to.[1]

As for substitutions for some of the other major allergens, there are a number of options available to you as more and more companies are creating products with food allergies in mind. This is very evident if you walk down the aisles of your local supermarket. If you have a milk allergy, you will notice that there are a number of different "milks" available to you that are derived from soy, almond, or rice and do not contain milk. If you have a wheat allergy and are looking to substitute something for wheat flour, you have a few options available to you such as potato flour, rice flour, or garbanzo bean flour. These examples are by no means all inclusive and are meant as general guidelines. If you go to the Food Allergy Research & Education website (www.foodallergy.org) or Kids with Food Allergies' website (www.kidswithfoodallergies.org), both offer a lot of great recipes from members. You can also connect with these members through the organization's social media pages and even share information or recipes that you may have discovered for yourself. Additionally, there are many cookbooks available now that are completely devoted to those who suffer from food allergies. After some trial and error, you may find that you would like to create your own cookbook filled with recipes. Cooking food-allergy friendly meals will not be just beneficial to you, but they can be enjoyable for the whole family, which is exactly what happened for Mark L. and his family.

Mark is a twin and often jokes that he wished his twin could take half of his allergies. Mark's twin brother does not have any allergies, but this has not stopped either of them from cooking allergy-friendly food for the whole family to enjoy. The twins' first experience with cooking came from attending a summer camp where the boys were told they had a choice of picking a class to take. Mark thought that taking a cooking class would be a lot of fun, but because of his allergies, there was some discussion on whether this would be feasible.[2] Luckily, Mark's counselor was also one of the cooking teachers. She spoke with the other cooking teacher, Alison S., to ask what could be done.

Alison had never dealt with allergies before, but was completely on board. Her thought was that summer camp should be about having fun and discovering new opportunities or abilities, so she starting modifying and redeveloping recipes to teach all of the campers. Alison was inspired by Mark and his desire to cook despite being allergic to so many foods, and she continued to keep in contact with Mark and his family by offering cooking classes. Through these cooking classes, Alison was able to create a larger support system for Mark and his family. It was important for Alison to teach that no matter what special dietary needs a person may have, preparing and eating food does not need to be a source of frustration; rather, it should be viewed as exciting to see how recipes can be modified. In fact, Alison admits that some of her favorite foods to prepare came from recipes that were modified for Mark and his family.[3]

Any kind of food can be fair game to make as long as ingredients are modified or substituted. The following are some recipes that come from personal ones that my mother, sister, and I have created. They use simple ingredients and are not too involved for you to begin your cooking journey. If you find you cannot have some of the ingredients, then feel free to substitute or to modify them to make them your own and safe to eat.

Recipes

Guacamole Dip

Ingredients:

- 2 avocados
- 1 tomato
- 1 small red onion
- 1 teaspoon garlic powder or 3 cloves of minced garlic
- Lemon
- Lime
- Salt
- Pepper

Directions:

Scoop avocado into a mixing bowl, making sure it is mashed.
Chop up the red onion and mix into the avocados.
Add a teaspoon of garlic powder or the chopped cloves of garlic (whichever you prefer).
Stir mixture together and add lemon juice, lime juice, salt, and pepper to taste.
Serve with bread, pita chips, or tortilla chips of your choice.

Focaccia Bread

Ingredients:

- 2 cups of flour (your choice of flour)
- 1/2 cup of cold water
- 1 tablespoon of olive oil
- 1 tablespoon of melted butter (use butter substitute if need be)
- Pecorino Romano cheese to sprinkle (substitute with a cheese alternative if need be)

Directions:

Preheat oven to 450 degrees.

Pour the flour and water into a large mixing bowl and stir vigorously. You should start to notice the mixture taking on a more dough-like appearance.

Knead the dough into a ball and make a well (small indent) in the middle of the ball of dough.

Add the olive oil in the well and begin to knead the dough again, forming another ball.

Roll out the dough into a thin layer and spread onto a baking sheet. Brush the melted butter onto the dough and sprinkle the Pecorino Romano cheese to your liking.

Bake on the top rack of the oven for 8–10 minutes or until lightly golden brown.

Simple Meat Sauce

Ingredients:

- 1 28-ounce can of Pastene Kitchen Ready Tomatoes
- 1 pound of ground beef or ground turkey
- 2 teaspoons of salt
- 3 cloves of garlic
- 1 cup of water
- 2 1/2–3 tablespoons of olive oil (enough to drizzle over the beef or turkey)

Directions:

Drizzle 1 tablespoon of olive oil to coat the bottom of the saucepan.

Take the ground beef or ground turkey and put into the saucepan.

Chop up the garlic cloves and mix into the ground beef or turkey.

Mix in the salt and drizzle the rest of the olive oil over the ground beef or turkey.

Sauté the beef or turkey until mostly cooked and then add the can of tomatoes. (Save the can.) Let it come to a simmer for a few minutes.

Fill the can with water and add to the saucepan.

Cook on low for 1–1 1/2 hours.

Stuffed Shells

Ingredients:

- Simple meat sauce (or any tomato sauce of your choice)
- 1 box of large pasta shells
- 2 teaspoons of salt
- 1 15-ounce container of ricotta cheese (substitute with a cheese alternative if need be)
- 1 cup shredded mozzarella (substitute with soy or nondairy cheese if need be)
- Romano cheese to taste (omit if need be)

Directions:

Preheat oven to 350 degrees.

Boil shells according to box directions.

In a large bowl, add the container of ricotta cheese, the package of shredded cheese, and salt, and mix together. Stuff each shell with cheese mixture.

In a baking pan, pour tomato sauce so it lightly coats the pan.

Place the stuffed shells with cheese mixture into the baking pan. Pour sauce in and on top of each shell.

Cover with aluminum foil and bake in the oven for roughly 20 minutes.

Top with Romano cheese when ready to serve.

Stuffed Meatballs

Ingredients:

- 1 pound of ground beef
- 3/4 cup of grated Romano cheese (substitute with a cheese alternative if need be)
- 1/2 cup of bread crumbs (substitute rice or potato bread crumbs if need be)
- 2 teaspoons of salt
- Cubed cheddar cheese (substitute with a cheese alternative if need be)

Directions:

Preheat oven to 350 degrees.

Mix all of the ingredients together except the cubed cheddar cheese.

Form the mixture into balls, being sure to add water as needed to moisten the mixture.

Make a hole in the center of the meatballs that you are forming and place the cubed cheese in the center. Roll into balls again and place on a baking sheet.

Bake in the oven for approximately 30 minutes or until the cheese is melted in the middle of the meatball and the meat is cooked through. Feel free to top with tomato sauce before baking as well.

Orange Chicken

Ingredients:

- 1–2 pounds of chicken cutlets (or 1–2 pounds boneless chicken breasts, cut into smaller pieces)
- 3 broccoli crowns
- 1–2 cloves of garlic
- 2 teaspoons of salt
- 2 1/2–3 tablespoons of olive oil
- 2 cups of orange juice

Directions:

Put the chicken into a small sauce pan and sprinkle with 1 teaspoon of salt. Lightly cook on low.

When the chicken has been seared, pour the 2 cups of orange juice over the chicken and use more orange juice if need be to cover the chicken completely. Bring to a rolling boil.

Wash the broccoli crowns and cut apart to put into a separate pan.

Chop up the garlic and stir into broccoli with olive oil and 1 teaspoon of salt. Sauté the broccoli with a fork until tender.

Cook 2 cups of white or brown rice according to box directions.

The chicken will be done when the orange juice has reduced to make a sticky coating (usually 20–30 minutes).

Mix in the sautéed broccoli and pour over the rice.

Breaded Chicken Cutlets

Ingredients:

- 2 pounds of chicken cutlets
- 2 lemons
- 2 cloves of garlic
- 1 tablespoon of fresh parsley finely chopped
- 2 cups of olive oil (1 cup for marinade and 1 cup for frying)
- 1/2 teaspoon of salt
- 1/2 cup of plain bread crumbs (substitute rice or potato bread crumbs if need be)
- 1 cup of grated Romano cheese (use cheese substitute if need be)

Directions:

Combine juice of 2 fresh lemons and 1 cup of olive oil for marinade. Add chicken and chill overnight in dish or plastic bag.

Combine bread crumbs, Romano cheese, finely chopped garlic, finely chopped parsley, and salt in a mix to coat the chicken.

Take chicken out of the fridge and submerge the cutlets into the bread-crumb mix, making sure to coat both sides.

Heat 1/2 cup of oil in a frying pan adding more oil as needed. Add bread crumbs to the pan and heat on medium until the crumbs sizzle.

Fry the cutlets until golden brown on each side.

Chicken, Cheese, and Broccoli Rollups

Ingredients:

- 1–2 pounds of chicken cutlets
- 3 broccoli crowns
- 2 teaspoons of kosher salt
- 1 cup shredded cheddar cheese (use cheese substitute if need be)
- 1 tablespoon of olive oil
- 1/2 cup of bread crumbs (use rice or potato bread crumbs if need be)
- 1/2 cup of Romano cheese (use cheese substitute if need be)

Directions:

Preheat oven to 350 degrees.

Boil or steam the broccoli crowns.

Pound out both sides of the chicken cutlets to make them thin. Sprinkle both sides with kosher salt.

Lay the cutlets flat in a baking dish, putting the broccoli in the center and sprinkle with cheddar cheese.

Roll the cutlets with the seam on the bottom of the pan (you may use a toothpick to keep them closed if need be).

Generously sprinkle the Romano cheese, then the bread crumbs. Drizzle olive oil over the cutlets, but use sparingly.

Bake for approximately 20 minutes or until the chicken is cooked through.

Shepherd's Pie a La Jessica

Ingredients:

- 5 pounds of white or yellow potatoes
- 3 pounds of ground beef
- 2 ears of fresh corn
- 1 14.5-ounce can of diced tomatoes
- 2 cloves of garlic
- 1/4 cup of olive oil
- 2 teaspoons of salt
- 1 cup of shredded cheddar cheese (use cheese substitute if need be)
- ½ cup of milk (use milk substitute if need be)
- 1 stick of butter (use butter substitute if need be)
- 1 pound of ground beef or ground turkey

Directions:

Boil the potatoes until tender. Add milk, butter, and 1 teaspoon of salt or more to taste and mash. Then set aside.

Boil two ears of corn and cool.

In a frying pan, add enough oil to lightly cook the garlic until it becomes translucent.

Add the ground beef and 1 teaspoon of salt. Cook the ground beef until it is no longer red, drain the water/oil from the ground beef, and set aside.

Put the ground beef in a large casserole dish sprinkling the cheddar cheese over the ground beef. Layer the diced tomatoes, corn, and top with the mashed potatoes.

Bake in the oven at 350 degrees until the cheese melts and potatoes have a light brown crust. You may also add slabs of butter to the top of the mashed potatoes to avoid dryness.

Grandma's Italian Wedding Cookies

Ingredients:

- 1/2 cup of unsalted butter (use butter substitute if need be)
- 1 3/4 cup of confectioner's sugar
- 3/4 teaspoon of salt
- 3 1/2 teaspoons of vanilla extract (use more or less depending on prefer-ence)
- 3 cups of sifted, all-purpose flour (use flour of your choice)
- 1 cup of Enjoy Life Foods Semi-Sweet Chocolate Mini Chips

Directions:

Preheat the oven to 325 degrees.

Cream the butter and slowly mix in the other ingredients, but be sure to reserve 1 cup of confectioner's sugar. As you continue to mix the ingredients, it should become fluffy.

Using a teaspoon, take the cookie mixture and roll into a ball. Once you have formed the cookie, place in an ungreased baking/cookie sheet.

Bake in the oven for approximately 20–30 minutes, being careful not to brown the cookies. When the cookies are finished baking, allow to cool for about 10 minutes.

Take the reserved confectioner's sugar and roll the cookies into the sugar. Place in a separate dish and the cookies will be ready to serve.

The next few recipes come from Kat S., fourteen years old, and founder of TeenFAAB (Teen Food Allergy and Anti-Bullying). Kat is a perfect example of coming into her own when dealing with her food allergies and becoming not only a self-advocate, but an advocate for others as well. She started her website (www .teenfaab.com) when she was in the sixth grade, and it grew from there. In addition to posting recipes to her website, Kat is also featured on TeenFAAB's www

.youtube.com channel in "Cooking with Kat" episodes where you can see first-hand how delicious food-allergy friendly recipes can be.[4]

Homemade Pancake Mix

Source: www.unsophisticook.com

Ingredients:

- 6 cups all-purpose flour, sifted
- 3 tablespoons of baking powder
- 1 tablespoon salt
- 1/2 cup of cold unsalted dairy-free margarine

Directions:

Measure the sifted flour, baking powder, and salt into a large bowl. Use a wire whisk to blend thoroughly.

Cut in cold margarine using a pastry cutter until thoroughly incorporated.

Store refrigerated in an airtight container for up to four months.

Apple Kat

Kat's own food allergy-friendly version of Apple Betty

Ingredients:

- 2 cups of thinly sliced apples
- 2 tablespoons of orange juice
- 1/4 cup and 2 tablespoons of all-purpose flour
- 1/2 cup white sugar
- 1/4 teaspoon of ground cinnamon
- 1/2 pinch of salt
- 1/4 cup of dairy-free margarine

Directions:

Preheat the oven to 375 degrees.

Lightly grease the pie plate.

Mound sliced apples in the pie plate. Sprinkle with orange juice.

In a medium bowl, mix the flour, sugar, cinnamon, and salt. Cut in the dairy-free margarine until the mixture resembles coarse crumbs. Scatter over the apples.

Bake in preheated oven for 45 minutes. Serve warm and hope you enjoy!

Kat's Applesauce Oatmeal Muffins

Ingredients:

- 1 1/2 cups of oats, uncooked, old fashioned
- 1 1/4 cups of flour
- 3/4 teaspoon cinnamon
- 1 teaspoon baking powder
- 3/4 teaspoon baking soda
- 1 cup unsweetened applesauce
- 1/2 cup soy milk
- 1/2 cup packed brown sugar
- 1 cup of dairy-free yogurt (e.g., coconut yogurt or soy yogurt)
- 3 tablespoons oil

Directions:

Preheat oven to 400 degrees.

Combine all dry ingredients.

Add the remaining ingredients. Mix just until dry ingredients are moistened.

Grease bottom of muffin tins or use paper muffin cups.

Fill muffin cups almost full.

Bake 20–22 minutes or until golden brown. Serve warm.

Cooking with Kat

In addition to her cooking and running TeenFAAB, Kat also participates in many allergy groups, including FARE (Food Allergy Research & Education) and FAACT (Food Allergy & Anaphylaxis Connection Team). She is on the Teen Advisory Council for both organizations. As a member of the council, she completes monthly projects such as questionnaires, and in November of 2013, Kat even presented at the National Teen Summit for FARE regarding food allergies and antibullying and how it can be negatively portrayed in the media. Kat wishes to continue to spread food allergy awareness, education, and tolerance through her own website and the organizations she is a member of. When asked what teenagers should know specifically or keep in mind with regard to living with food allergies, Kat had this to say:

> It is better to remain safe than sorry. People have lost their lives due to anaphylaxis and taking chances with foods with "May contain" statements. Never take chances—that can be fatal. Always read ingredients and don't eat foods that do not have a label at parties or other social events. Always remember to look beyond the downside of allergies and look at them in a "FAABulous" way. Because of food allergies I have become a stronger and more efficient person. Food allergies may have made my life challenging, but they have also made it better. If I didn't have allergies I wouldn't be educating others and I would not be making a difference in the world. It is an honor being part of the food allergy community and to be a part of something so special.[5]

Living Well

The food allergy community is indeed something special. You can find a great deal of support and many resources by joining groups such as FARE, FAACT, and the Asthma and Allergy Association of America. By becoming a member of these groups or following them through social media outlets, you can connect with other teenagers who understand what you are going through or who can provide guidance on what works for them. There are special programs and events that you can attend and meet other teens in person and continue to expand your world and make it your own. You may also find that by connecting with other teens, you want to become more of an advocate yourself. Maybe you want to start your own group in your area or at your school, or create your very own website or blog dealing with food allergies. If you do not find a calling to do one of these things, that's OK, too. Just know that you have support and guidance available to you.

Living with allergies can be difficult and certainly frustrating at times. Some days will be easier than others, but do not let this stop you in any aspect of your life. Remember that there is always an alternative way to do something. Look at a frustrating situation from a different perspective. What works for some people with regard to their food allergies may not be a good option for others with food allergies. Although it may not be easy, trust me when I tell you that you will be able to make the necessary adjustments to work with the challenges that sometimes arise when living with food allergies. Also, as many teenagers interviewed for this book have mentioned, allergies have not been all bad. There are many things you can gain as a result of having food allergies. Emily H., eighteen years old and a FARE Teen Advisor, had this to say when talking about how she has dealt with her food allergies over the years:

When I was in middle school I had a tough time with my peanut allergy. I denied its existence because it made me different from my friends. In high school I realized that being different is okay and realistically, I'm not even all that different; I just have to take a few extra precautions around the food table at events and also at restaurants. It's not a big deal! Anyway, knowing my unhappiness, I wanted to make other people happier and have better middle school and high school experiences than me. I wanted to give them some support and a sympathetic ear to listen. As a Teen Advisor for FARE, I've sent in numerous allergy-safe recipes and have posted many times in the Facebook group both asking questions and answering them! The FARE Facebook group is really a great resource for teenagers with allergies and I highly recommend joining it for anyone who might be on the fence.

I certainly go out to eat at restaurants and knock on wood, have always had a great experience. My typical order is a hamburger and French fries, but sometimes I branch out to chicken fingers, mozzarella sticks, pizza, or a turkey club sandwich. If anything is to be unsafe, it is usually the hamburger bun or another bakery bread product. In that case, my mom or I will literally bring a bun to the restaurant and I will order a bun-less burger and fries. If the French fries are fried in peanut oil or cross-contaminated somehow, I can usually request baked fries; the chef will cut slices of potato and put them on a baking sheet and just bake them plain. They're delicious! Sometimes the breading of the chicken isn't safe or the bread of the turkey club isn't safe, but there are almost always other options. My mom or I will usually ask the waiter or waitress to bring the manager or head chef out, and he or she is typically very helpful, often willing to make my meal themselves in a completely separate part of the kitchen with clean equipment. Knock on wood, I have never come across a restaurant that couldn't feed me . . . but I also stay away from known allergy-unfriendly places!

Because of Irish Dance, I've been to Ireland twice and Scotland once for various World Championships. Because of my college search, I've been on more planes in the past two years than normal. My allergies have never stopped me from traveling. Since I have had to fly relatively often, I usually take the first flight out of the airport, often at 6 in the morning. That is when the plane is the cleanest, as the planes are cleaned overnight but not between flights. I once took a plane at 11 pm and that was a really bad idea because there were peanut shells everywhere. Anyway, my mom typically puts the peanut allergy disclaimer on my boarding pass when she purchases the tickets. When I get to the airport, I tell the staff at the terminal about my allergy and they give me a pass to preboard, so I can wipe down my seat with wipes, wearing plastic gloves just in case. Once on the plane, I also remind the flight attendants about my allergy. Knock on wood, I've never been told that they are required to or for some reason must serve peanuts on the flight. However, I do my research before I fly to make sure that the airline I am using will be willing to not serve peanuts on their flights. My family and I stick to chain restaurants when we travel; I've been to over 10 Hard Rock Cafes across the United States and Europe! Yes, only going to chain restaurants takes away from the "international cuisine" appeal of traveling abroad. However, I would much rather stay out of the hospital than try haggis and corned beef. At restaurants in Europe especially, my mom or I will explain my allergy, the wait staff will bring out the manager and he/she will almost always accommodate me in some way. Often, before we leave our house, my mom will call or e-mail a few restaurants in the area to ask if they can accommodate peanut allergies, so we know upon arrival of a few places that are safe. We travel just like anyone else, touring all the landmarks and enjoying our time abroad. However, it just takes a little bit of extra planning ahead of time to make sure that there are restaurants that I can eat at. We also always pack an entire suitcase of food, including chips and crackers but also pasta and sauce and the ingredients of various meals; we stay at either an apartment or a condo or a hotel room with a kitchen so my mom can cook our meals, particularly our breakfasts and dinners, with the food we packed. We also check online for local supermarkets and so after landing in the country we can stock our new kitchen! All it takes is a little extra planning. Allergies have never stopped me from traveling!

I carry my EpiPen with me at all times in addition to Benadryl tablets. Before each school year, my mom makes multiple kits of EpiPens and Benadryls to pack in various bags. I have one of these kits in my Irish Dance bag, one in my wristlet that I carry everywhere, one in my track bag (it stays on the field with me when we're running), and I have a giant kit with multiple EpiPens and a whole container of Benadryl in my school nurse's office. I would say about 75 percent of my family knows how to use an EpiPen. The other 25 percent of the family lives too far away and we don't see them very often. At family events, I'm always near my mom or dad or brother anyway and they certainly know how to use an EpiPen. All of my close friends—either from cross-country and track, Irish Dance, or school—who I spend all my time with know how to use an EpiPen. I've trained them during downtime at practices or in class. Cross-country and track meets and practices often involve PowerBars and other protein bars that are typically contaminated. I have found my own replacement bars (they're by the brand Promax and my favorite flavor is chocolate chip cookie dough!) and I'm sure they're just as good. When my friends eat their PowerBars or other peanut-y bars, they just wash their hands right after eating. They're really good about keeping me safe and I really appreciate it! The same thing happens in Irish Dance. As soon as I joined the cross-country/track teams and my Irish Dance school, I didn't really talk about my allergy, figuring there was no need to mention it until the food came out. At that point, I told all of my newfound friends about the severity of my peanut allergy, the precautions they could take, and how to use an EpiPen. They all absolutely agreed to wash their hands and thanked me for telling them.

The one piece of advice that I would give to any teenager dealing with food allergies is not to be afraid to tell people about your allergies. I know I struggled with that in middle school but thinking back, that was just me being stupid. Food allergies are a part of you but they don't define you. You have to tell your friends, boyfriend/girlfriend, friends' parents, teachers, coaches, administrators, restaurant managers, waiters, waitresses, airplane flight attendants, and other people to keep yourself safe. Food allergies are real and they are scary, but they don't have to be as long as you take precautions.[6]

Like Emily, you too will find that as you get older, you will learn the best way to deal with your food allergies and that there may even be some positives that come out of it. The following are a few quotes from those teenagers who were interviewed discussing the challenges of having food allergies as well as important things to keep in mind.

Don't let having food allergies embarrass you. There is nothing to be embarrassed about and it's important for others to know about it. That is the only way that you can stay safe.—Colton C.[7]

A piece of advice I would give to a teenager dealing with food allergies is that it's okay to relax—just don't take risks. You don't have to be nervous about it, but you shouldn't do things that would be unsafe such as eating unknown foods. Of course, you probably know that already.—Natalie L.[8]

I think a teenager dealing with food allergies should know that it shouldn't stop them from having fun and living their life. Surround yourself with people who are willing to listen, accommodate, and understand you and your food allergies.—Kayla S.[9]

Have a plan in place in case you do have an allergic reaction. Talk to your classes at the beginning of the school year and let them know about you and your allergies, how they can help you and others to stay safe.—Haley R.[10]

If you are allergic to nuts and are going to any type of sporting event, I highly recommend wearing closed-toed shoes. There are nuts everywhere and it makes me uncomfortable to be around a place with nuts all over the floor wearing flip-flops.—Katie O.[11]

My friends, most teachers, and cafeteria workers are all aware of my food allergies and the cafeteria has a no-nut policy. In case of an emergency I carry two epinephrine auto-injectors with me at all times in addition to those present in the nurse's office. I am currently a high school senior in the process of applying to college. Almost all of the colleges I have looked at have students with food allergies and make sure to take the necessary precautions and exhibit flexibility to meet students' needs. Ultimately, however, I am responsible for keeping myself safe and healthy and I am confident that sixteen years of attentiveness and caution will serve me well.—Aarush G.[12]

Growing up with allergies has had some positives. It has made me able to connect with people and to become more empathetic and able to connect with people. I never feel alone. My friends have been supportive either by not eating foods I am allergic to when I am around and my neighborhood friends do not even have the offending foods in their house. Every cloud has a silver lining.—J. F.[13]

Having food allergies has given me more successes than downfalls. It may seem hard, but people are out there who understand and who can help. You are not alone and there is nothing to be afraid of. There are certain challenges to having allergies, but it is nothing to be embarrassed about. Your allergies will become natural to you, all your friends should know about it and it won't even be a "thing" anymore.—Brett N.[14]

Remember to always keep those lines of calm-munication open regarding your food allergies. Trust in your family, friends, doctors, and the rest of those important people within your circle who make up your food allergy crew. If something is bothering you, speak up and do not let it fester. Most disagreements stem from a misunderstanding or from a lack of communication. You have been taught how to manage your allergies and can continue to use these same practices as you get older, but never be afraid to try and improve a situation. You can use each moment as a teachable moment, if not for other people, then for yourself. Allergies are a part of your life, but they are not what makes up your entire life.

It Happened to Me:
A Note from the Author about Life with Food Allergies

Adapting to and dealing with food allergies on your own can sometimes seem like a monumental task, but remember that you always have control over how you deal with a situation. When I became more vocal about my food allergies, I noticed that there was a difference between the way I viewed my allergies (since I developed them later on in life and was not diagnosed until the age of twenty-one) and the way friends who had allergies since birth viewed living with their respective food allergies. An example of this was when I was seated next to a friend with a milk allergy while at an engagement party for one of our mutual friends. The food looked absolutely amazing and it was a full sit-down, four-course meal. Neither one of us were eating the food because of the risk of a reaction, and it was not a big deal as we had both eaten before the party and brought safe foods. However, I saw the usual glances and questioning eyes from other party attendees, wondering why neither one of us had a plate in front of us. Then one of the hosts of the party approached our table. I took a deep breath ready to explain about food allergies, when my friend seated next to me took the lead and answered for both of us. While I was getting anxious about the conversation that did not even occur yet, in less than a matter of minutes, he had explained that we both had food allergies and the meal looked wonderful, but we could not eat it. The host felt bad and proceeded to say that there must be some special food that she could provide us. My friend explained the problem of cross-contamination and it was not a big deal because we were there to celebrate the engagement of our mutual friend and quickly led the conversation in another direction. Sitting there, I realized it really was not a big deal and I was creating a problem and needless anxiety for no reason. Food allergies will always be a part of you, but they are manageable and you will still be able to live a fulfilling life.

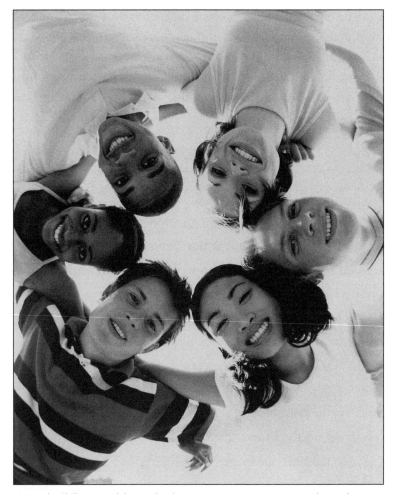

Keep building and broadening your support network and open up your world with great people surrounding you. You can do this!

You have so many great qualities that are uniquely yours. So if life seems to give you lemons, make lemonade. If you are allergic to the lemonade, then use those unique skills and qualities of yours to make a different kind, one that no one has ever tried, and share it with the world!

Congratulations! You are well on your way to becoming more independent and to leading a fulfilling life with food allergies. Never forget that you have a large network and support system available to you.

Glossary

allergist: a specialist in the diagnosis and treatment of allergies, asthma, and immune deficiency disorders; also known as an immunologist.

allergy/allergic reaction: a medical condition that causes someone to have an abnormal immune response after eating, touching, or breathing something that is harmless to most people.

anaphylaxis: a serious allergic reaction involving multiple systems of the body.

antibody: a blood protein produced in response to and counteracting a specific antigen.

antigen: any substance that can stimulate the production of antibodies and combine with them.

antihistamine: drug used to counteract the histamine productions in allergic reactions.

anxiety: a fear or nervousness about what might happen.

asthma: a condition in which your airways narrow and swell and produce extra mucus. This can make breathing difficult and trigger coughing, wheezing, and shortness of breath.

auto-injector: a device used to deliver a single dose of medication.

biopsy: the removal of tissue, cells, or fluids from the body in order to check for illness or disease.

celiac disease: an autoimmune disorder in which the body attacks itself in the presence of gluten, damaging the lining of the small intestine.

cross-contact/cross-contamination: when proteins from one food are accidentally mixed with proteins from another food.

cross-reactivity: when the immune system mistakes one antigen for another. For instance, cross-reactivity is typically seen in oral allergy syndrome when the immune system mistakes the pollen in pitted fruits for the pollen in birch trees.

desensitization: a method that is sometimes used to allow people to tolerate greater amounts of an allergen before they suffer a reaction.

eczema: an inflammatory condition of the skin characterized by redness, itching, and oozing vesicular lesions that become scaly, crusted, or hardened.

eosinophilic esophagitis: an allergic inflammatory condition of the esophagus that involves eosinophils, a type of white blood cell.

epinephrine: also known as adrenaline. It is a hormone that is secreted by the adrenal glands and is currently the only medication that can be used to stop an allergic reaction.

food allergy: an abnormal immune system response to certain foods.

food intolerance/sensitivity: an abnormal reaction to food involving the digestive system; not IgE mediated.

gluten: a protein that is found in wheat, barley, and rye.

immune system: the bodily system that protects the body from foreign substances, cells, and tissues.

immunoglobulin E (IgE): a type of antibody that is present in minute amounts in the body but plays a major role in allergic diseases. IgE binds to allergens and triggers the release of substances from mast cells that can cause inflammation.

oral allergy syndrome: an allergic reaction to certain raw fruits and vegetables.

Notes

Introduction

a. Food Allergy Research & Education, "Facts and Statistics," www.foodallergy.org/facts-and -stats? (accessed October 4, 2014).
b. TargetStudy, "Adrenaline," targetstudy.com/knowledge/invention/179/adrenaline.html (accessed October 4, 2014).
c. Allergic Living, "Food Allergy: Discovery Channel Airs Food Allergy Documentary," *Allergic Living*, allergicliving.com/2013/09/04/discovery-channel-to-air-food-allergy-documentary/ (accessed November 22, 2014).

Chapter 1

1. National Institute of Allergy and Infectious Diseases (NIAID), "What Is Food Allergy?" www.niaid.nih.gov/topics/foodAllergy/understanding/Pages/whatIsIt.aspx (accessed October 4, 2014).
2. NIAID, "Guidelines for the Diagnosis and Management of Food Allergy in the United States," NIH Publication No. 11-7699, May 2011.
3. Centers for Disease Control and Prevention (CDC), "Food Allergies in Schools," www.cdc .gov/healthyyouth/foodallergies/ (accessed October 4, 2014).
4. CDC, "Voluntary Guidelines for Managing Food Allergies in Schools and Early Care and Education Programs," www.cdc.gov/healthyyouth/foodallergies/pdf/Food_Allergy_Guide lines_FAQs.pdf (accessed October 4, 2014).
5. Food Allergy Research & Education (FARE), "About Anaphylaxis," www.foodallergy.org/ anaphylaxis (accessed October 4, 2014).
6. FARE, "Epinephrine Auto-injectors," www.foodallergy.org/treating-an-allergic-reaction/ epinephrine (accessed November 16, 2014).
7. American College of Allergy, Asthma, and Immunology, "Food Allergy Testing," www.acaai .org/allergist/allergies/Types/food-allergies/Pages/food-allergy-testing.aspx (accessed October 4, 2014).
8. U.S. Food and Drug Administration, "Important Issues for Allergen-Specific IgE Testing," www.fda.gov/MedicalDevices/Safety/AlertsandNotices/TipsandArticlesonDeviceSafety/ ucm109367.htm (accessed October 4, 2014).
9. Asthma and Allergy Foundation of America (AAFA), "Oral Allergy Syndrome," www.aafa .org/display.cfm?id=9&sub=20&cont=728 (accessed October 4, 2014).
10. NIAID, "Oral Allergy Syndrome and Exercise-Induced Food Allergy," www.niaid.nih.gov/ topics/foodAllergy/understanding/Pages/OASExercise-inducedFA.aspx (accessed October 4, 2014).
11. Dr. David Stukus, e-mail interview with author, February 9, 2014.

12. AAFA, "IGE's Role in Allergic Asthma," www.aafa.org/display.cfm?id=8&sub=16&cont=54 (accessed November 2, 2014).

13. FARE, "Know the Difference: Milk Allergy vs. Dairy Allergy vs. Lactose Intolerance," *FARE Blog*, October 11, 2014, blog.foodallergy.org/2014/10/11/know-the-difference-milk -allergy-vs-dairy-allergy-vs-lactose-intolerance/ (accessed October 11, 2014).

14. Stukus, e-mail interview.

15. National Institute of Diabetes and Digestive and Kidney Diseases, "Celiac Disease," digestive.niddk.nih.gov/ddiseases/pubs/celiac/ (accessed October 4, 2014).

---

a. AchooAllergy.com, "A History or Allergies and Asthma, Part One: The Ancients' Perspective," www.achooallergy.com/history-allergies.asp (accessed October 4, 2014).

b. AchooAllergy.com, "A History or Allergies and Asthma, Part One."

c. CDC, "CDC Study Finds 3 Million U.S. Children have Food or Digestive Allergies" (press release), www.cdc.gov/media/pressrel/2008/r081022.htm (accessed October 4, 2014).

d. FARE, "Avoiding Cross-Contact," www.foodallergy.org/tools-and-resources/managing-food -allergies/cross-contact? (accessed October 4, 2014).

e. Kids with Food Allergies Foundation, "Conditions Related to Food Allergies," Facebook page, June 18, 2011.

f. David M. Fleischer et al., "The Sublingual Immunotherapy for Peanut Allergy: A Randomized Double-Blind, Placebo-Controlled Multicenter Trial," *Journal of Allergy and Clinical Immunology* 1, no. 1 (January 2013): 15–21.

g. "Celebs with Food Allergies and Sensitivities" (slideshow), *Huffington Post*, www.huffington post.com/2013/05/23/worst-gluten-free-mistakes_n_3246820.html (accessed October 4, 2014).

Chapter 2

1. Centers for Disease Control and Prevention, "Food Allergies in Schools," www.cdc.gov/ healthyyouth/foodallergies/ (accessed October 4, 2014).

2. Food Allergy Research & Education, "Facts and Statistics," www.foodallergy.org/facts-and -stats? (accessed November 29, 2013).

---

a. Dennis Hevesi, "George Rieveschl; Invented Benadryl," *Boston.com*, September 30, 2007, www.boston.com/news/globe/obituaries/articles/2007/09/30/george_rieveschl_invented_ benadryl/ (accessed October 4, 2014).

b. Spencer, quoted in Food Allergy Research & Education, "Teen Talk—Food Allergies," YouTube video, www.youtube.com/watch?v=lMcZuMtoA-Y (accessed October 4, 2014).

c. EpiPen, www.epipen.com (accessed October 4, 2014).

d. Alex, quoted in Food Allergy Research & Education, "Teen Talk—Food Allergies," YouTube video, www.youtube.com/watch?v=lMcZuMtoA-Y (accessed October 4, 2014).

Chapter 3

a. Gracien L., "Nut Allergies Take Schools by Storm," *Teen Ink*, www.teenink.com/opinion/all/ article/549835/Nut-Allergies-Take-Schools-by-Storm/ (accessed October 4, 2014).

b.   Alex, quoted in Food Allery Research & Education, "Teen Talk—Food Allergies," YouTube video, www.youtube.com/watch?v=lMcZuMtoA-Y (accessed October 4, 2014).

c.   Katie L., "Bad Nuts," *Teen Ink*, www.teenink.com/hot_topics/health/article/4681/Bad-Nuts/ (accessed October 4, 2014).

Chapter 4

1.   Tiffani P., e-mail interview with author, September 13, 2014.

2.   Heidi S., e-mail interview with author, September 9, 2014.

3.   U.S. Department of Health and Human Services, "What Is Bullying? Bullying Definition," Stopbullying.gov, www.stopbullying.gov/what-is-bullying/definition/index.html (accessed October 4, 2014).

4.   Eyal Shemesh, Rachel A. Annunziato, Michael A. Ambrose, Noga L. Ravid, Chloe Mullarkey, Melissa Rubes, Kelley Chuang, Mati Sicherer, and Scott H. Sicherer, "Child and Parental Reports of Bullying in a Consecutive Sample of Children with Food Allergy," *Pediatrics* 131, no. 1 (January 2013): e10–17.

5.   Food Allergy Research & Education, "Spread the Word about Food Allergy Bullying," www.foodallergy.org/its-not-a-joke/share#.VBSw3PldWSo (accessed October 4, 2014).

6.   Dr. David Stukus, e-mail interview with author, February 9, 2014.

a.   Lee Phillips, "Teenage Stress," *Teen Ink*, www.teenink.com/hot_topics/health/article/297707/Teenage-Stress/ (accessed October 4, 2014).

b.   Spencer, quoted on Food Allergy Research & Education, "Teen Talk—Food Allergies," YouTube video, www.youtube.com/watch?v=lMcZuMtoA-Y (accessed October 4, 2014).

c.   Michelle G., e-mail interview with author, September 13, 2014.

d.   Jake H., e-mail interview with author, September 16, 2014.

Chapter 5

1.   Alex N., e-mail interview with author, September 9, 2014.

2.   U.S. Department of Health and Human Services, *The Surgeon General's Call to Action to Prevent and Reduce Underage Drinking* (Rockville, MD: U.S. Department of Health and Human Services, 2007), www.ncbi.nlm.nih.gov/books/NBK44364/ (accessed October 12, 2014).

3.   Office of Juvenile Justice and Delinquency Prevention, *Drinking in America: Myths, Realities, and Prevention Policy* (Washington, DC: U.S. Department of Justice, Office of Justice Programs, Office of Juvenile Justice and Delinquency Prevention, 2005).

4.   U.S. Department of Health and Human Services, *The Surgeon General's Call.*

5.   Tim Mainardi, "Tired of Morning Hangovers? You Could Be Allergic to Alcohol," *Huffington Post*, April 15, 2014, www.huffingtonpost.com/dr-tim-mainardi-/alcohol-allergies_b_4769469.html (accessed October 12, 2014).

a.   Katie O., e-mail interview with author, September 25, 2014.

b.   Zoe P., e-mail interview with author, September 4, 2014.

c.   Kayla S., e-mail interview with author, September 15, 2014.

d.   Emily C., e-mail interview with author, September 10, 2014.

Chapter 6

1. Centers for Disease Control and Prevention (CDC), *Voluntary Guidelines for Managing Food Allergies in Schools and Early Care and Education Programs Frequently Asked Questions*, www .cdc.gov/healthyyouth/foodallergies/pdf/Food_Allergy_Guidelines_FAQs.pdf (accessed October 4, 2014).
2. CDC, *Voluntary Guidelines for Managing Food Allergies.*
3. Dr. David Stukus, e-mail interview with author, February 9, 2014.
4. Food Allergy Research & Education, "About Us," www.foodallergy.org/about (accessed October 4, 2014).
5. Food Allergy & Anaphylaxis Connection Team, "About FAACT," www.foodallergyawareness .org/about/ (accessed October 4, 2014).
6. Stukus, e-mail interview.
7. Kristin Beltaos, e-mail interview with author, April 29, 2014.
8. Sloane Miller, e-mail interview with author, September 1, 2014.
9. Miller, e-mail interview.
10. Miller, e-mail interview.
11. Miller, e-mail interview.

a. Ruth Lovett-Smith, phone interview with author, August 11, 2014.
b. "Celebs with Food Allergies," *ABC News*, abcnews.go.com/Health/Allergies/photos/celebs -food-allergies-17923373/image-18030675 (accessed October 4, 2014).

Chapter 7

1. Jennifer M. Maloney, Martin D. Chapman, and Scott H. Sicherer. "Peanut Allergen Exposure through Saliva: Assessment and Interventions to Reduce Exposure," *Journal of Allergy and Clinical Immunology* 118, no. 3 (2006): 719–24. See more at www.kidswithfoodallergies.org/ resourcespre.php?id=18#sthash.KWZ5CNbR.dpuf (accessed October 4, 2014).
2. "Dating with Food Allergies, a Tricky Business," *Allergic Living*, allergicliving.com/2010/07/ 02/food-allergy-celiac-dating-kissing-issues/2/ (accessed October 4, 2014).

Chapter 8

1. ServSafe, "FAQ," www.servsafe.com/allergens/faqs#2 (accessed October 4, 2014).
2. National Restaurant Association, "National Food Safety Month to Focus on Food Allergies," September 4, 2013, www.restaurant.org/News-Research/News/National-Food-Safety-Month-to-focus-on-food-allerg (accessed October 4, 2014).
3. Sarah Klein, "The 15 Most Allergy-Friendly Restaurant Chains," *Huffington Post*, March 29, 2014, www.huffingtonpost.com/2014/03/29/food-allergies-restaurant-chains_n_5051227. html (accessed October 4, 2014).

a. Zoe P., e-mail interview with author, September 4, 2014.

b. Olger Enger, "Local Teen Inspired Bill to Make Restaurants Safer," *Newport Patch*, May 18, 2012, patch.com/rhode-island/newport/local-teen-inspired-bill-to-make-restaurants-safer#.VDCEBPldWSp (accessed October 4, 2014).

c. AllergyEats, "The AllergyEats 2014 List of Most Allergy-Friendly Restaurant Chains," *Food for Thought* (blog), March 14, 2014, www.allergyeats.com/blog/index.php/the-allergyeats-2014-list-of-most-allergy-friendly-restaurant-chains/ (accessed November 16, 2014).

d. Emily C., e-mail interview with author, September 10, 2014.

Chapter 9

1. Theresa E. Sommers, "Travel Insurance, Travel Health Insurance, & Medical Evacuation Insurance," Centers for Disease Control and Prevention, wwwnc.cdc.gov/travel/yellowbook/2014/chapter-2-the-pre-travel-consultation/travel-insurance-travel-health-insurance-and-medical-evacuation-insurance (accessed October 4, 2014).

2. Walt Disney World, "Special Dietary Requests," disneyworld.disney.go.com/guest-services/special-dietary-requests/ (accessed October 4, 2014).

3. Mylan, "Mylan Signs Strategic Alliance Agreement with Walt Disney Parks and Resorts to Enhance Access to EpiPen® (Epinephrine) Auto-Injectors," November 7, 2014, www.mylan.com/news/press-releases/item?id=123258 (accessed November 16, 2014).

4. Thomas Faddegan, "How to Cruise with Food Allergies," Cruiseline, December 26, 2013, cruiseline.com/bonvoyage/before-you-cruise/what-to-know/how-to-cruise-with-food-allergies (accessed October 4, 2014).

5. U.S. Department of Transportation, "Management of Passengers Who May Be Allergic to Allergens," December 31, 2002, Advisory Circular Number 121-36, www.faa.gov/documentLibrary/media/Advisory_Circular/AC121-36.pdf (accessed October 4, 2014).

6. Kids with Food Allergies, a Division of Asthma and Allergy Foundation of America, "Flying with Food Allergies: Medical and Legal Concerns" (webinar), June 17, 2014.

7. U.S. Department of Justice, Civil Rights Division, Disability Rights Section, "Questions and Answers about the Lesley University Agreement, and Potential Implications for Individuals with Food Allergies," ADA.gov, www.ada.gov/q&a_lesley_university.htm (accessed October 19, 2014).

8. Kimberly A. Pierce, RDN, LDN, interview with author, February 17, 2014.

9. Pierce, interview.

10. Pierce, interview.

11. Beth Winthrop MS, RD, CNSC, "Managing Food Allergies in a Campus Setting," *Tastings*, Fall 2013.

12. Asthma and Allergy Foundation of America, New England Chapter, "Food Allergies and College: Planning for Campus Life," September 21, 2011.

13. Mackenzie G., e-mail interview with author, September 26, 2014.

a. Norwegian Cruise Line, "Accessibility Assistance," www.ncl.com/about/accessible-cruising (accessed November 16, 2014).

b. Carnival Cruise Lines, "Guests with Disabilities," www.carnival.com/about-carnival/special-needs/dietary-needs.aspx (accessed November 16, 2014).

c. Disney Cruise Line, "Guests with Disabilities," disneycruise.disney.go.com/ships-activities/ships/services/guests-with-disabilities/ (accessed November 16, 2014).

d. Royal Caribbean International, "Frequently Asked Questions," www.royalcaribbean.com/customersupport/faq/details.do?pagename=frequently_asked_questions&pnav=5&pnav=2&faqSubjectName=Health+%26+Safety&faqId=322&faqSubjectId=335&faqType=faq (accessed November 16, 2014).

e. American Airlines, "Special Meals and Nut Allergies," www.aa.com/i18n/travelInformation/duringFlight/dining/special-meals.jsp (accessed November 17, 2014).

f. Delta Airlines, "Peanut Allergy Policy," www.delta.com/content/www/en_US/agency/useful-resources/peanut-allergy-policy.html (accessed November 17, 2014).

g. JetBlue Airlines, "Allergies," help.jetblue.com/SRVS/CGI-BIN/webisapi.dll/,/?St=166,E=0000000000180152242,K=7154,Sxi=2,t=casePrint,case=obj(3071) (accessed November 17, 2014).

h. Southwest Airlines, "Customers with Disabilities," www.southwest.com/html/customer-service/unique-travel-needs/customers-with-disabilities-pol.html (accessed November 17, 2014).

i. United Airlines, "Customers with Peanut Allergies," www.united.com/web/en-US/content/travel/specialneeds/needs/peanut-allergies.aspx (accessed November 17, 2014).

j. Ryan M., "Let's Go to College with Food Allergies," *Teen Ink*, teenink.com/college_guide/college_essays/article/45290/Lets-Go-to-College-with-Food-Allergies/ (accessed October 4, 2014).

Chapter 10

1. U.S. Food and Drug Administration (FDA), "Have Food Allergies? Read the Label," www.fda.gov/forconsumers/consumerupdates/ucm254504.htm (accessed October 4, 2014).

2. Mayo Clinic Staff, "Food Allergies: Understanding Food Labels," Mayo Clinic, www.mayoclinic.org/diseases-conditions/food-allergy/in-depth/food-allergies/art-20045949?pg=1 (accessed October 4, 2014).

3. FDA, "Food Allergen Labeling and Consumer Protection Act of 2004 Questions and Answers," December 12, 2005, updated July 18, 2006, www.fda.gov/Food/GuidanceRegulation/GuidanceDocumentsRegulatoryInformation/Allergens/ucm106890.htm (accessed February 3, 2015).

4. Claire Gagne, "How to Read a Label When You Have Food Allergies," *Allergic Living*, January 6, 2014, allergicliving.com/2014/01/06/how-to-read-a-label-when-you-have-food-allergies/ (accessed February 3, 2015).

5. Margaret Morrison, "'Hypoallergenic' Cosmetics," *FDA Consumer*, April 1978, www.fda.gov/cosmetics/labeling/claims/ucm2005203.htm (accessed October 4, 2014).

6. U.S. Department of Agriculture, Plants Database, "Peanut," plants.usda.gov/core/profile?symbol=ARHY (accessed October 4, 2014).

a. FDA, "Guidance for Industry: Questions and Answers Regarding Food Allergens, Including the Food Allergen Labeling and Consumer Protection Act of 2004 (Edition 4); Final Guidance," October 2006, www.fda.gov/food/guidanceregulation/guidancedocumentsregulatoryinformation/allergens/ucm059116.htm (accessed October 4, 2014).

Chapter 11

1. "Basic Recipe Substitutions for People with Egg Allergy," May 2013, www.kidswithfood allergies.org/resourcespre.php?id=104 (accessed October 4, 2014).
2. Mark L., phone interview with author, February 9, 2014 .
3. Alison S., phone interview with author, February 20, 2014.
4. Kat S., e-mail interview with author, April 7, 2014.
5. Kat S., e-mail interview with author, April 7, 2014.
6. Emily H., e-mail interview with author, September 13, 2014.
7. Colton C., e-mail interview with author, September 14, 2014.
8. Natalie L., e-mail interview with author, September 13, 2014.
9. Kayla S., e-mail interview with author, September 15, 2014.
10. Haley R., e-mail interview with author, September 16, 2014.
11. Katie O., e-mail interview with author, September 25, 2014.
12. Aarush G., e-mail interview with author, September 27, 2014.
13. J. F., e-mail interview with author, February 16, 2014.
14. Brett N., phone interview with author, February 9, 2014.

Food Allergy Resources for Teens

The following is a list of resources that you may find useful along your journey to living well with food allergies. Please note that this is by no means an all-inclusive list of all resources available to you, but it will be a great starting point. Feel free to add to this list any time you want and share with others.

Organizations

AllergyHome
Website: www.allergyhome.org
E-mail: use the contact form on the website
Twitter: @AllergyHome_org

Anaphylaxis Canada
2005 Sheppard Avenue East
Suite 800
Toronto, Ontario M2J 5B4
Canada
Main phone number: (866) 785-5660
E-mail: info@anaphylaxis.ca
Website: www.anaphylaxis.ca
Special website for teens: www.whyriskit.ca
Twitter: @AnaphylaxisCAN

Asthma and Allergy Foundation of America
8201 Corporate Drive
Suite 1000
Landover, MD 20785
Toll-free phone number: (800) 727-8462
E-mail: info@aafa.org
Website: www.aafa.org
Twitter: @AAFANational

Food Allergy & Anaphylaxis Connection Team (FAACT)
P.O. Box 511

West Chester, OH 45071
Main phone number: (513) 342-1293
Fax number: (513) 342-1239
E-mail: info@foodallergyawareness.org
Website: www.foodallergyawareness.org
Twitter: @faactnews

Food Allergy Research & Education (FARE)
National Headquarters
7925 Jones Branch Drive
Suite 100
McLean, VA 22102
Toll-free phone number: (800) 929-4040
Fax number: (703) 691-2713
E-mail: Use the contact form on the website
Website: www.foodallergy.org
Twitter: @FoodAllergy

Kids with Food Allergies, a Division of the Asthma and Allergy Foundation of
    America
5049 Swamp Road
P.O. Box 554
Fountainville, PA 18923
Main phone number: (215) 230-5394
Fax number: (215) 340-7674
Website: www.kidswithfoodallergies.org
Twitter: @kfatweets

Food Allergy Coaches

Kristin Beltaos, MA
Website: www.agiftofmiles.com

Sloane Miller
Website: www.allergicgirl.com

Magazines

Allergic Living magazine
P.O. Box 1042

Niagra Falls, NY 14304
Main phone number: (888) 771-7747
E-mail: info@allergicliving.com
Website: www.allergicliving.com
Twitter: @AllergicLiving

Living Without's Gluten Free & More magazine
535 Connecticut Avenue
Norwalk, CT 06856
Toll-free phone number: (800) 474-8614
Website: www.glutenfreeandmore.com
Twitter: @Living_Without

Delight Gluten Free magazine
Toll-free phone number: (800) 305-6964
E-mail: info@delightglutenfree.com
Website: www.delightglutenfree.com
Twitter: @delightgfmag

Cookbooks

What's to Eat? The Milk-Free, Egg-Free, Nut-Free Food Allergy Cookbook. Author: Linda Marienhoff Coss.
The Allergy Free Pantry. Author: Colette Martin.
The Food Allergy Mama's Baking Book: Great Dairy, Egg, and Nut Free Treats for the Whole Family. Author: Kelly Rudnicki.
Allergen-Free Baker's Handbook. Author: Cybele Pascal.
Allergy-Free and Easy Cooking. Author: Cybele Pascal.

Books Dealing with Food Allergies

A Little Bit Can Hurt: The Shocking Truth about Food Allergies—Why We Should Care, What We Can Do. Author: Donna T. DeCosta, MD.
Food Allergies: A Complete Guide for Eating When Your Life Depends on It. Author: Scott H. Sicherer.
Allergic Girl: Adventures in Living Well with Food Allergies. Author: Sloane Miller.
Don't Kill the Birthday Girl: Tales from an Allergic Life. Author: Sandra Beasley.
Food Allergies for Dummies. Author: Robert A. Wood, MD. Contributor: Joe Kraynak.

Living with Life-Threatening Food Allergies: A Teenager's Guide to Doing It Well. Author: Elisa Stavola.

Manufacturer Websites for Auto-Injectors

Not only do these websites provide information about the actual auto-injector that each respective pharmaceutical company makes, but they also provide additional resources for those with allergies. If you take a look at each website, you will find information on anaphylaxis, how the epinephrine works, and other resources for those with allergies. Be sure to check it out.

www.epipen.com (produced by Mylan)
www.auvi-q.com (produced by Sanofi)

Websites of Companies That Offer Medical Identification Jewelry and/or Carrying Cases for Auto-injectors

www.allerbling.com
www.hopepaige.com
www.myidsquare.com
www.allergyapparel.com
www.carrynine.com
www.bluebearaware.com
www.epi-essentials.com
www.omaxcare.com (particularly good for athletes)

Music about Food Allergies

Musician and food allergy educator, Kyle Dine (www.kyledine.com)

Websites to Food-Allergy-Friendly Products

www.beanfieldssnacks.com
www.divvies.com
www.enjoylifefoods.com
www.jenniferswaybakery.com
www.iansnaturalfoods.com
www.paschachocolate.com

www.peanutfreeplanet.com
www.premiumchocolatiers.com
www.serenityfoods.com
www.sodeliciousdairyfree.com
www.sunbutter.com
www.suncups.com
www.udisglutenfree.com
www.vermontnutfree.com
www.wowbutter.com

Other Helpful Websites

nuttiesforachange.wix.com/nfac
www.allergyeats.com
www.anaphylaxis101.com
www.bestallergysites.com
www.freedible.com
www.glutendude.com
www.snacksafely.com
www.teenfaab.com

Index

504 plan 65, 68, 76, 78
1986 Air Carrier Access Act 109

AAA 103
action plan(s) 64, 68
Adrenaclick 5
Alavert 21
allergic reaction 52, 3, 4, 5, 6, 7, 8, 9, 10, 11, 13, 17, 19, 20, 21, 22, 25, 30, 32, 33, 35, 36, 37, 38, 39, 43, 52, 53, 55, 56, 59, 60, 64, 65, 66, 69, 72, 77, 78, 79, 84, 86, 88, 91, 95, 103, 104, 406, 109, 110, 121, 122, 123, 125, 144, 147, 148
allergist 5, 6, 7, 8, 9, 13, 14, 26, 31, 32, 65, 68, 69, 70, 71, 72, 73, 75, 76, 81, 102, 103, 121, 147, 149
allergy 1, 2, 3, 4, 6, 7, 8, 9, 10, 11, 12, 13, 14, 15, 19, 20, 22, 23, 24, 25, 26, 27, 30, 31, 32, 33, 37, 39, 43, 45, 48, 49, 50, 51, 52, 53, 54, 57, 58, 59, 60, 62, 64, 65, 68, 71, 72, 73, , 75, 76, 77, 78, 79, 80, 82, 84, 86, 87, 88, 90, 92, 94, 95, 96, 97, 98, 104, 106, 107, 111, 112, 114, 116, 117, 120, 121, 122, 126, 127, 128, 129, 130, 137, 138, 139, 140, 141, 142, 143, 144, 145, 147, 148, 149
AllergyEats 73, 94, 97, 98
American Express 103
Americans with Disabilities Act 64, 113, 149
anaphylaxis 4, 5, 6, 8, 9, 13, 14, 19, 22, 25, 36, 50, 54, 55, 57, 60, 65, 78, 79, 140, 149, 167
antibody 2, 3, 10, 147
antibullying 137, 139
antigen 147

antihistamine 20, 21, 147
anxiety 33, 34, 36, 37, 38, 62, 66, 70, 76, 79, 81, 82, 104, 108, 145, 147
asthma 9, 15, 79, 140, 147
auto-injector 5, 6, 9, 84, 88, 112, 147
Auvi-Q 5, 147

Beltaos, Kristin 76
Benadryl 20, 21, 54, 124, 142
Best Allergy Sites 72
biopsy 12, 147
bullying 47, 48, 49, 50, 78, 137, 139, 147

Carnival Cruise Line 107, 147
celiac disease 10, 11, 12, 13, 14, 15, 27, 96, 113, 114, 147
Centers for Disease Control 15, 63, 147
chef cards 95, 103, 147
Cherrybrook Kitchen 58
college 13, 21, 30, 67, 113, 114, 115, 116, 117, 127, 141, 144, 147
Cooking with Kat 138, 139
cross-contact/cross-contamination 8, 13, 22, 33, 36, 57, 59, 78, 88, 91, 94, 95, 96, 108, 112, 116, 121, 128, 147
cross-reactivity 8
cruise 106, 107, 108

dairy 10, 62, 80, 94, 133, 138, 139
Delta Air Lines 111
desensitization 9, 147
disability 64, 147
Disney 105, 106, 107
divvies 58
doctor 6, 8, 9, 11, 13, 14, 31, 64, 65, 67, 68, 69, 70, 71, 72, 73, 74, 75, 76, 81, 101, 102, 103, 109, 112, 144

eczema 4, 9, 79, 147
egg 3, 10, 36, 39, 60, 66, 80, 86, 120, 121, 126, 129
Enjoy Life Foods 58, 106, 137
eosinophilic esophagitis 9, 147
epinephrine 5, 6, 9, 20, 21, 22, 30, 54, 55, 106, 109, 144, 147
EpiPen 5, 21, 23, 53, 54, 55, 65, 106, 123, 142, 143, 147
Esposito, Jennifer 11

Facebook 74, 75, 141
family 1, 15, 19, 25, 29, 30, 31, 32, 33, 34, 35, 36, 37, 38, 39, 40, 41, 51, 52, 53, 55, 62, 63, 65, 66, 67, 68, 77, 79, 80, 81, 82, 91, 96, 101, 103, 104, 108, 121, 127, 130, 142, 144
Federal Aviation Administration 109
fish 3, 60, 79, 80, 93, 120, 121
food allergy 3, 4, 5, 6, 7, 9, 12, 13, 14, 15, 20, 30, 32, 33, 39, 45, 48, 49, 50, 53, 54, 62, 97, 98, 107, 114, 116, 117, 120, 121, 129, 130, 137, 138, 140, 144
Food Allergy & Anaphylaxis Connection Team 74, 75, 139, 140
food allergy coaches 76, 79
Food Allergy Research Education 45, 48, 49, 54, 74, 75, 95, 96, 117, 139, 140, 141
food intolerance/sensitivity 9, 10, 12, 14
Food Safety Modernization Act of 2011 63

general practitioner 68
gluten 10, 11, 12, 73, 96, 113, 114, 147

health maintenance organizations 71
Hitch 20
hotel 55, 104, 105, 106, 108, 142
hypoallergenic 122, 125, 126

immune system 2, 3, 7, 8, 10, 11, 12
immunoglobulin E 2, 10

Individual Health Plan 76, 77
insurance 70, 102, 103

JetBlue 111

Kids with Food Allergies 9, 49, 130

Lesley University 113, 114
lifestyle 17, 50, 62, 81

Mabel's Labels 129
mast cells 10
Miller, Sloane 79, 82
milk 3, 8, 10, 22, 60, 66, 86, 90, 93, 98, 120, 126, 129, 130, 136, 139, 145
Mylan 106

Norwegian Cruise Line 107
Nutties for a Change 45

oral allergy syndrome 7, 8, 147

Pascha Chocolates 58
peanut 3, 9, 13, 22, 24, 39, 40, 45, 46, 54, 56, 57, 80, 87, 108, 109, 111, 120, 126, 141, 142, 143
pediatrician 67, 68, 75
Pinterest 75
pollen 8
preventative care 70

restaurants 23, 32, 40, 41, 50, 53, 55, 60, 61, 62, 66, 73, 79, 84, 88, 91, 92, 93, 94, 95, 96, 97, 98, 99, 105, 106, 107, 126, 127, 141
roommate 113, 115
Royal Caribbean International 107

shellfish 3, 80, 93, 120, 121
Skeeter Snacks 111
skin prick test 6, 7
Smartphone Apps 73
social media 71, 72, 74, 75, 76, 130, 140

Southwest Airlines 111
soy 3, 66, 86, 93, 120, 122, 123, 130, 133, 139
Stonehill College 114
Stukus, Dr. David 9, 11, 12, 49, 72, 75
support group 30, 32, 74, 75, 116
symptoms 3, 4, 5, 6, 8, 10, 11, 12, 14, 19, 21, 25, 38, 56, 60, 64, 69, 73, 88, 115

Teen Advisor 54, 139, 141
travel 30, 55, 79, 95, 96, 98, 101, 102, 103, 104, 105, 107, 108, 109, 110, 112, 113, 127, 141, 142

tree nut 3, 22, 24, 45, 79, 80, 93, 101, 108, 111, 120, 125, 126
Twitter 75

U.S. Department of State 103
U.S. Department of Transportation 109
United Airlines 111
university 9, 20, 113, 114

Vermont Nut Free 58
villas 104, 106, 112

well visits 70
wheat 3, 10, 11, 12, 60, 66, 80, 120, 122, 130

About the Author

Jessica Reino is a children's book author who was diagnosed with multiple life-threatening food allergies at the age of twenty-one, although she began exhibiting symptoms as a teenager. She is very active in the food allergy community and is a member of the Asthma and Allergy Foundation of America New England Chapter, the Food Allergy & Anaphylaxis Connection Team, as well as Food Allergy Research & Education. When Jessica is not spreading food allergy awareness, she enjoys spending time with family and friends and developing new works within children's literature. She is a member of the Society of Children's Book Writers and Illustrators and is represented by Sadler Children's Literary. Connect with Jessica on her author website (www.jessicareino.com) or follow Jessica on Twitter (@JNRlitauthor).